MIND FOOD & SMART PILLS

MIND FOOD
&
SMART PILLS

*A Sourcebook for the
Vitamins, Herbs, and Drugs
That Can Increase Intelligence,
Improve Memory, and
Prevent Brain Aging*

Ross Pelton, R.Ph., Ph.D.
with Taffy Clarke Pelton

DOUBLEDAY
NEW YORK   LONDON   TORONTO   SYDNEY   AUCKLAND

PUBLISHED BY DOUBLEDAY
A division of Bantam Doubleday Dell Publishing Group, Inc.
666 Fifth Avenue, New York, New York 10103

DOUBLEDAY and the portrayal of an anchor with a dolphin
are trademarks of Doubleday, a division of Bantam Doubleday
Dell Publishing Group, Inc.

Drawings on pages 26 and 27 by Jackie Aher

Library of Congress Cataloging-in-Publication Data
Pelton, Ross.
Mind food and smart pills : a sourcebook for the
vitamins, herbs, and drugs that can increase
intelligence, improve memory, and
prevent brain aging / Ross Pelton,
with Taffy Clarke Pelton.—1st ed.
     p.   cm.
   Bibliography: p.
   ISBN 0-385-26138-1
   1. Intellect—Nutritional aspects.
2. Neuropharmacology.   3. Brain—Aging—Prevention.
I. Pelton, Taffy Clarke.   II.   Title.
QP398.P44   1989   89-1513
153.9—dc20   CIP

Contents

A Note from the Authors

The information presented in this book is based on research that has been published and is available to anyone. My role has been to collect and organize a vast amount of information that has for the most part appeared only in scientific journals and publications, and to present it in such a way that it is understandable to the general public.

To the best of my knowledge, substances described in this book adhere to two main principles. First, the effects are well researched and documented. Second, they are safe and non-toxic.

I believe that the information in this book is extremely important to both individuals and society. I want to stress the following points:

1. At no point in this book do I recommend that anyone take or try any of the nutrients or drugs about which I have written. My purpose is to present information, not to diagnose, prescribe, or suggest that anyone start taking anything.

2. I strongly recommend that anyone who is interested in taking any of the nutrients or drugs in this book do so under the guidance of a qualified health professional.

3. The research reported in this book is interpreted and presented as accurately as possible. However, I am not infallible and conclusions from research are not always correct. Do not assume that the research reported herein is the last word on the subject.

4. Adequate long-term studies have not been done in many of the areas reported and much of the work must still be regarded as experimental. This is another important reason to exercise caution and seek advice from a qualified health professional before using any of the drugs, nutrients, or herbs described in this book.

5. Because of differences in individual biochemistry, optimal levels for a drug or nutrient can vary as much as one thousand times from one person to the next. Again, exercise caution and seek guidance from a qualified health professional.

6. I do not have any financial involvement with any of the products, manufacturers, or suppliers mentioned or recommended in this book.

7. Children, pregnant women, and individuals with existing medical conditions should not experiment with any of the drugs, nutrients, or herbs in this book.

Remember, use caution, common sense, and seek the advice of a qualified health professional before acting on any of the information contained in this book.

Foreword

One of the most common complaints from many of my new patients is that their memory is not as sharp as it used to be. I hear this not only from the elderly, but from college-age and middle-age patients as well. Clearly, with the information explosion and increased sensory overload to which we are increasingly exposed, memory sharpness and increased thinking ability become more important to all of us.

In *Mind Food & Smart Pills*, Dr. Ross Pelton describes how our brain works, and tells us what we can do to improve its performance. He describes a variety of nontoxic drugs and nutrients that have demonstrated efficacy in improving mental functioning, alleviating depression, fighting "brain fatigue," and even improving sexual performance.

Many of these substances can be obtained without a prescription in a health food store. Others must be prescribed by a physician. Some of the newer, most effective brain-enhancing drugs are not yet approved in the United States, and must be imported from other countries. Fortunately, the FDA had recently loosened its restrictions against the importation of unapproved drugs and such substances may now be legally imported into the United States for personal use. Dr. Pelton gives several sources to obtain such drugs in his book.

I frequently prescribe many of these substances for my patients, usually with gratifyingly positive results.

Mind Food & Smart Pills is obviously not just another

popular health book. It is a well-researched, meticulously referenced compendium of nutrients, drugs, and herbs that favorably influence the brain and mental processes. It should be read by anyone who could benefit from improved memory, more accurate thinking, and faster data acquisition and processing. Physicians who treat patients with memory disorders or who are interested in preventive medicine will benefit from this book, as it contains a great deal of information that is not readily available elsewhere.

Ward Dean, M.D., M.S.
The Center for Bio-Gerontology
Thousand Oaks, California

I

MIND FOOD
&
SMART PILLS

1
Introduction

The greatest gift that we humans have is our intelligence. We value intelligence so highly that most people consider only good health to be of greater importance. We are beginning to understand that intelligence is primarily learned, not bred. The "art" of becoming intelligent requires an appreciation of the fact that we can develop our intellectual abilities through sensorimotor exercises, mental exercises, an enriched environment, improved overall health, optimal nutrition, and new drugs that increase and preserve mental powers.

Exciting breakthroughs in scientific research are giving us a new understanding of human intelligence. Scientists now believe that the limits of our intelligence are not rigidly set in our brains at conception or birth. Human intelligence can be developed!

This book discusses certain nutrients and drugs that can increase human intelligence and prevent much of the deterioration usually associated with aging, such as senility.

The effects of these nutrients and drugs can be grouped in two categories: enhancement of intelligence and maintenance of intelligence.

The enhancement of intelligence is the most startling result of using the information contained in this book. Significant improvement in mental performance and memory can be produced by some of the drugs discussed here. However, the benefits for "normal" people are measurable, but usually not dramatic. Many people perform better on tests of intellectual functioning without feeling any more intelligent.

There is no special sensation or feeling associated with improved mental performance. We perform better and like the results without knowing why. When there is a lack in performance due to nutritional deficiencies or brain aging, the change is more noticeable. In those cases the person really feels the difference. The most dramatic observable increases in intelligence are seen in older people with mild to moderate senility.

The ability to increase intelligence is a goal that naturally excites people. However, the maintenance of intelligence is of equal if not greater importance. Whereas enhancement means getting smarter, maintenance means not getting dumber. Maintenance is the prevention of brain aging. One of the saddest spectacles in our society is the aged person who has lost the ability to remember, to think, and even to carry out the simplest of tasks. Anything that can help to prevent such tragedy is of immeasurable value. By preventing damage to brain cells, certain drugs and nutrients can prevent senility and brain aging. Some of the agents discussed in this book can actually reverse part of the damage that has been done.

There are two ways in which nutrients and drugs promote optimal functioning of the brain. First, they give the brain adequate supplies of oxygen and certain biological building blocks so it can maintain a high energy level and store memories. Second, they protect the brain against damage from chemical poisons in our environment. The obvious conclusion is that the functioning of the brain is greatly affected by our diet and the supplements that we take.

It is worth emphasizing that the prescription drugs discussed in this book have a high degree of safety and are considered to be without serious side effects.

Why Take Mind Food and Smart Pills?

What can you realistically expect to achieve by embarking on a personal program of intelligence-enhancing drugs and nutrients? The health and biochemical uniqueness of each individual varies so much that the best approach is to set a range of possible results. Those who suffer from mild to moderate impairment of brain function will tend to notice more dramatic improvements because they have more symptoms to serve as a basis for judging rehabilitation.

Those who are closer to optimal brain function may not be as aware of the improvements in intelligence and mental abilities as those who suffer from some degree of impairment. Some of the effects that frequently occur are:

An increase in mental energy
Greater ability to concentrate
Longer periods of high-level mental ability
Greater ease in memorizing material
More alertness with less sleep

Taking the nutrients and drugs discussed in this book will not make you a genius, but you can expect to make the most of the mental abilities you have.

The nutrients and drugs discussed in this book are also able to reverse some aspects of the aging process. Those who are suffering from the early stages of senility, who have suffered certain types of brain damage, or who have decreased mental ability resulting from drug abuse may notice dramatic changes in mental ability and functioning.

Those who have achieved an improved level of mental functioning as a result of this program can expect to maintain a high level of mental performance and retard the gradual loss of intelligence associated with aging. Remember, the correction of a problem is much more noticeable than its prevention.

Myths That Limit Human Potential

There are three major myths related to health and intelligence that contribute to a general misunderstanding of the capacity we have to increase our intelligence and to maintain optimal mental functioning.

Myth 1: The Myth of a Fixed Intelligence. Most people believe that we are born with a fixed level of intelligence, and that is our lot in life. This is a myth. Exciting new research is showing that both the brain and human intelligence are capable of being developed. There are genetic differences, but we are now learning that environmental factors may be far more important.

A great deal of scientific research that documents the ability to increase intelligence will be presented in subsequent chapters of this book.

Myth 2: The Myth of a Healthy Diet. Nutritional supplements are important because the average life style and environment exposes us to far greater levels of toxins than ever before, and the average American diet, high in processed and fast foods, is nutritionally deficient.

In the last four decades, developed countries (with the United States leading the way) have switched from an agricultural food supply to an industrial food supply. Industrial farming techniques have greatly increased the level of toxins in our food and water supply. At the same time the nutritional quality of commercially grown foods has declined over the past several decades. Today two thirds of the average American diet is highly processed "food."

Much of our commercial food supply is not nutritionally adequate and is a major contributor to chronic degenerative disease. Nutritional supplements are almost a necessity to any wellness-oriented life style.

Myth 3: The Myth of Aging. To understand aging we must understand the difference between chronological aging and biological aging. Chronological aging is simply the measurement of the passage of time. We will continue to have birthdays; the pages of the calendar will continue to turn.

Biological aging, however, is the gradual destruction of the human body. Most people believe that biological and chronological aging happen together. This is a myth. As we grow older with time, we do not have to destroy our bodies. In fact, we now know that biological aging can be slowed down, it can be stopped, and in some cases it can even be reversed.

Old age is not a time of life. It is a condition of the body. It is not time that ages the body, it is abuse that does.

—Herbert Shelton

The Information Gap

The research reported in this book on enhancing mental abilities and maintaining optimal intelligence is so amazing that people have difficulty believing it. I am frequently asked how these discoveries can be true without having gained widespread attention.

The main reasons why this important information has not been disseminated are the information explosion and the nature of scientific writing. Computers and new scientific technology are making phenomenal growth possible in all areas of science. Nowhere is this mind-boggling process more evident than in the biological sciences. Some experts say that we are doubling the total amount of information in these areas of science every five years!

Not only do we have to deal with the quantity and speed at which new information is generated, we also have to evaluate the relative importance of this new knowledge in order to use it.

Quantum leaps are being made in our understanding of the body and mind, especially in the areas of brain research and human intelligence.

The information explosion is happening so quickly we cannot keep up with it. New discoveries are being published in thousands of medical and scientific journals every month. But usable, understandable information is not getting to the people who need it. Valuable new knowledge about intelligence-enhancing drugs and antiaging research is available, and yet most people don't know this information is available or how and where to find it.

Generally speaking, scientists do not communicate well with the general public; they write in a style suited to scientific journals and publications. The technical style of their writing is almost a foreign language to nonscientific readers.

This is not meant to be a criticism of scientists. It is just an insight into the nature of the game. Scientists' careers are often dependent on getting published in scientific journals. They don't get paid to write for the general public, nor do they have the time to do it.

The Right to Be Intelligent

One progressive country has undertaken an impressive program to implement recent discoveries in the area of intelligence. Venezuela, under the direction of Minister of Intelligence Luis Machado, has mounted an ambitious program to increase the intelligence of that country's entire population of 16 million people. The program has been operating for over five years and is attracting international attention. Testing Machado's fundamental belief that intelligence is learned, not bred, may become one of the most important social experiments of this century.

Machado has incorporated the best programs from thinkers and educators around the world. The Venezuelan program consists of sensorimotor exercises for infant development, visual education for three-year-olds, a chess program for children from seven to nine years old, a program designed to help students achieve rapid proficiency in playing musical instruments, and a series of programs designed by educator Edward de Bono entitled *Learn to Think*. This program, which stresses creativity, is being presented to 1.2 million children ages nine to fourteen as well as to adults.

Minister Machado (who is also a poet) speaks articulately and eloquently on the importance of intelligence. The following piece is taken from his book entitled *The Right to Be Intelligent*.

Everyone has, simply by existing, a right to be intelligent.
And to be provided with a way to become consistently more intelligent.
This is a right that must be recognized and held sacred.
Above all, the necessary conditions for the exercise of this right must be available.

This is society's mission and the primary obligation of its leaders. All of them.
The task of building a new society cannot be completed according to a single ideological current.
It is too transcendent to be partial.
Political leaders are therefore the first who must shake off indifference.
History will not forgive them lost time.

Until now intelligence has been a privilege.
The last stronghold of privilege.
The most ill-distributed wealth on Earth.
The cause and foundation of the remaining privileges.
Intelligence is a synonym of power.
Meditation on intelligence is meditation on power.

The education we know mechanizes.
It destroys originality.
It ages.
The affirmation, "Every child is a genius," and the fact that
so few adults really are, makes the search to widen the case
against the present system unnecessary.
There is its unescapable condemnation.

In any circumstance, "stupidity" is a curable "disease."
It is not a situation to be endured with resignation; it is a
social problem that can be combatted.
No one can become Einstein.
It is absurd to even try.
But anyone can become himself.
And there is no reason why a person should be anything less
than Einstein.

Genius is rare because the means of becoming one has not
been made commonly available.
A "genius" ought not be seen as one endowed with extraor-
dinary faculties.
A genius is not a superman.
But a normal man or woman.
The rest of us are infranormal.
We are called to reach the genius level.
And, in the future, to surpass it.
Today's exception will be tomorrow's rule.
Intelligence is only natural.
Stupidity requires explanation.

The revolution of intelligence will happen without fail in all
countries of the world.
It will begin in the arms of all mothers.
The day mothers realize that they are the wellsprings of their

children's intelligence, that day and for that reason alone, the world will be changed forever.

Ideas change the conditions of people's lives.
Behind every event is an idea.
A truth sown in the minds of human beings sooner or later bears fruit.
Only revolutions in ideas are true revolutions.
Every historical confrontation has an ideological substratum.
First, ideologies change.
Then, realities.

Today a society of and for intelligence can be consciously and humanly planned.
This is not a theory; it is a reality that transforms.
It is as if the ground beneath our feet were opening out onto one of the great paths of history, the one leading to the integral development of human reason. In possession of more developed minds, people will be able to find within themselves the elements needed to build a new society.
What they construct will be their own work.
The change will not be based on a previously determined goal; it will be the natural and necessary fruit of a radical change in the nerve center of society—the intelligence of man.

Everyone has the right to be free.
And the right to be freer.
Respect for people's freedom means that they are permitted to exercise the freedom they possess.
That is not sufficient.
Freedom has to be augmented.
The human being can be freer by the perfection of his own

being, which is gained in the progressive actualization of all his faculties.

Freedom is all that is necessary

Everything is ours if freedom is left to us.[1]

Reprinted with permission from:
Luis Alberto Machado
The Right to Be Intelligent
Pergamon Press Ltd., 1980

2
The Neuron: The Basic Unit

The abilities to think, remember, act, and react are centered in the brain. To understand how drugs and nutrients act on memory and intelligence, we need to know some of the basics about how the brain is structured and how it operates. A review of present knowledge about the functioning of the brain and nervous system reveals that, although the study of the brain has advanced tremendously in the last twenty years, we still know relatively little about how we store and process information, or how we think and remember.

Even though our knowledge about the most important functions of the brain is limited, we know a great deal about the basic levels of biological activity in the nervous system. And it is on this basic level that drugs and nutrients have their most important effects. This means that there is important information available about how nutrients and drugs affect the functioning of the nervous system, despite the fact that we may not know exactly how the nervous system produces intelligence and stores memories.

The Neuron

Despite its small size, the brain is unbelievably complex. The brain consists of up to one hundred billion individual neurons. These neurons carry the bioelectric impulses that enable the brain to carry out its different functions. By understanding how the neurons work we will learn the properties of the basic unit of the nervous system.

A neuron is a specialized nerve cell that takes advantage of the fact that most cells have a difference in electrical charge on each side of the cell membrane. This difference is very small, about 75 millivolts (75 thousandths of a volt), but it is large when we consider how small a cell is. The neuron is structured so that it can detect small electrical currents and transmit those currents to other cells. It is the flow of these bioelectrical currents that determines the thought processes of the brain.

There are two electrical states of a neuron that matter, the resting potential and the action potential. The resting potential is the small charge described above. This resting potential is the result of an active biological pump in the cell wall that pushes positively charged atoms out of the cell while keeping negatively charged molecules inside. The result is that the inside of the cell has a negative resting potential of about -75 millivolts, which means that it is negatively charged relative to the outside of the cell.

When the neuron is stimulated at special sites called synapses, there is a sudden rise in electrical potential inside the cell, and the charges of the inner and outer cell are reversed. The charge inside the cell rises to about $+50$ millivolts. This electrical charge quickly spreads along the cell wall.

When the neuron is stimulated enough it sends an electrical charge along a long fiber called the axon. The charge traveling down the axon is called the action potential. The action potential causes the axon to communicate with other neurons. It is the capacity of the neuron suddenly to switch electrical charge and produce an action potential that is the basis of nerve activity. By looking at how the neuron is constructed, we will see how it uses the action potential to transmit information and communicate with other neurons.

The Structure of the Neuron

The neuron, like other cells, has a cell body with a nucleus. What is different is that it has long fibers called dendrites and axons extending from the cell body. Most nerve cells have a single axon and several dendrites. The dendrites are tree-like structures that receive signals from the ends of the axons. This sets the basic direction of information flow through neurons. The signal is received at the dendrites, sent through the cell body, and ignites an all-or-nothing signal when it reaches the base of the axon. This all-or-nothing signal travels to the end of the axon and transmits its information to the dendrites of the next cell.

The axon is often insulated by a sheath of specialized cells composed of myelin, which acts like the covering of a household electrical cord. The charge travels like a common electrical current through the insulated portion but is much faster.

When the speed of transmission matters, there is plenty of insulation on the axon. The axon can be very long, up to three feet or more. For example, the pressure sensors in the feet give information to a neuron with an axon that travels all the way to the spinal cord. Since the spinal cord and brain need information about pressure on the soles of the feet while we are walking, the axons of these neurons are heavily insulated. If the centers that control walking don't get that information quickly, it becomes very difficult to walk without falling down.

While we need rapid transmission of information from our feet in order to walk, we can get all the information we need about the state of the stomach from slow, uninsulated neurons. The nerves that transmit signals from the stomach are slow-acting because speed of transmission is not important to our survival.

The axon ends in small bulbs called synaptic terminals. These end bulbs connect with receptors on the dendrites of other neurons to form synaptic connections. At the connection there is a space called the synaptic cleft or junction. The signal is sent across the synaptic cleft by chemicals called neurotransmitters. These synapses are the center of action in the nervous system.

In Figure 1A, we see the components of a synaptic junction. The end bulb contains small, round vesicles that contain the neurotransmitter chemicals. A synapse is much more complicated than a simple spark junction. The electric current that arrives at a synapse causes some of the synaptic vesicles to move rapidly toward the membrane of the end bulb. When the vesicles arrive at the membrane they release their neurotransmitters into the synaptic junction. (See Figure 1B.)

The neurotransmitter travels across the junction where it is

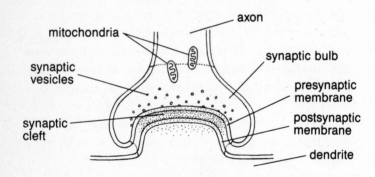

FIGURE 1A. Synaptic Junction of a Nerve Cell

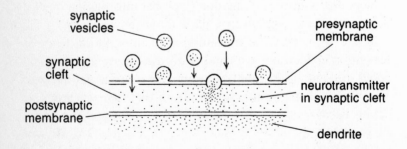

FIGURE 1B. Release of Neurotransmitter into Synaptic Cleft

taken up by receptors on the dendrite. This triggers a reaction in the receiving cell membrane and starts a current flowing. In this way nerve cells are able to communicate with each other and send signals from the body to the brain. The brain then processes those signals and sends out orders for action to the muscles and organs of the body.

The dendrites are the tree-like network of extensions that branch out from the body of the nerve cell. They form the network of pathways that allow brain cells to communicate with each other. A healthy neuron has a dendritic tree that branches into a network of hundreds of thousands of dendrites. The transmission of nerve impulses via dendritic pathways is also necessary for learning to take place. (See Figures 1A, 1B, and 2.)

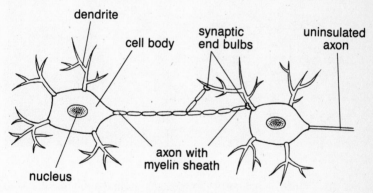

FIGURE 2. Structure of Nerve Cells

Dendrites are very fragile and easily damaged. The accumulated loss of dendrites interferes with communication between brain cells, bringing on symptoms of senility. Methods to prevent dendritic damage, the cause of the aging of the brain, will be a major point of focus in this book. Figures 3A, 3B, and 4 show the gradual destruction of the neuron with biological aging. The system of dendrites deteriorates, the axon shortens, and the cell body eventually withers away and dies. The brain depends on the complex system of connections between the dendrites and axons to function. As more and more brain cells are destroyed, intelligence decreases, and eventually the capacity to function as a human being disappears altogether.

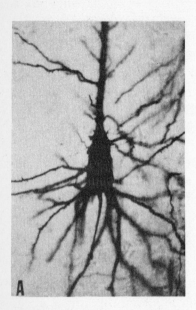 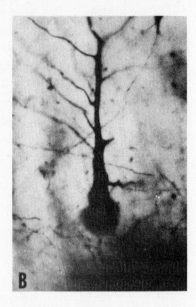

FIGURE 3A. Normal large cortical motor neuron in a young adult. Note the healthy dendritic system. FIGURE 3B. The same type of cell in a seventy-five-year-old individual. The massive change in the dendritic system is obvious. (Stained by Golgi method, X450.)

Courtesy of Dr. Arnold Scheibel, Department of Anatomy, University of California, Los Angeles.

The transmission of signals from one neuron to another seems like a simple process, but although we understand a great deal about the simplest level of this process—the nerve cell and synaptic junction—we know very little about the action of large numbers of neurons and how they process information. However, to understand how drugs and nutrients affect the nervous system, we need mainly to know about this simple level of nerve cell action. Nutrients and drugs have their major effect on this level. We can draw a parallel with muscular action. Basic muscle action depends on the contraction of muscle fibers. Poor nutrition deprives the muscle cells of the basic building blocks and vitamins that are necessary for good muscular action.

Good nutrition can ensure the best biological conditions for muscle growth and health, but it is practice that gets the muscles to work together. Nutrients work at the level of the individual muscle cell. Exercise stimulates cell growth and practice coordinates muscle activity. Without exercise, a good program of nutrition will produce only high-quality flab. Just working on strength training will produce larger, stronger muscles, but practice at the sport is necessary for developing coordination and smooth muscle action. Learning a sport like basketball involves the coordination of hundreds of muscles, requiring years of practice.

The same is true of the nervous system. Good nutrition essentially bathes the nerve cells in an optimal growth medium and enables them to perform at peak capacity. But if we do not use those cells, they will not develop and coordinate their activity to produce working intelligence. So it comes down to this—we may not know how nerve cells work together to produce intelligence, but we do know a good deal about how to take care of nerve cells so that it is possible to develop our intelligence to the greatest possible extent.

Chemical Actions at the Synaptic Junction

When the action potential arrives at the end bulb, it causes the synaptic vesicles to travel to the cell membrane and release their stores of neurotransmitter. There are several different kinds of neurotransmitter and new ones are being discovered daily. We will take a look at the most important ones.

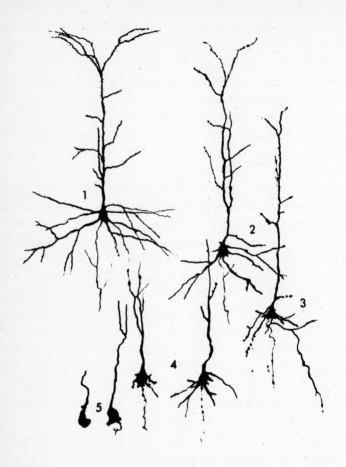

FIGURE 4. Series of large motor neurons tracing the course of degeneration from young, healthy adulthood (1) to an advanced demented state, as in Alzheimer's disease (5). (Drawings based on Golgi stained sections.)
Courtesy of Dr. Arnold Scheibel, Department of Anatomy, University of California, Los Angeles.

Acetylcholine. The most common neurotransmitter is acetylcholine. It travels across the synaptic cleft and arrives at receptors that begin the generation of current in the receiving cell.

After being used, the acetylcholine is broken down to acetate and choline to be taken up again by the end bulb. This breakdown is produced by an enzyme, acetylcholinesterase (AChE). Without the action of this enzyme the end bulb lacks enough of the basic building blocks of acetylcholine to prepare for the next signal it is to transmit.

After the end bulb has taken up new supplies of choline and acetyl, the mitochondria come into play. Each mitochondrion is a chemical factory that produces adenosine triphosphate (ATP). ATP is the major source of energy in cells. The mitochondria take glucose and oxygen and, through a complex chemical process called the citric acid cycle, they produce acetyl coenzyme A (acetyl CoA) and ATP. Then the acetyl CoA is combined with the choline molecule to produce acetylcholine.

To understand the importance of the process that turns acetate and choline back into acetylcholine we need to take a look at the brain's use of glucose and oxygen. The brain makes up only 2 percent of the body's weight, but it gets 15 percent of the blood supply. From this massive blood flow it extracts glucose and oxygen.

Most of the body's tissues can use proteins and fats as well as glucose as a source of energy. But the brain uses glucose exclusively as its source of energy—except under extreme conditions, such as starvation. The brain cells also consume great amounts of oxygen to metabolize this glucose.

The brain uses seven to ten times as much glucose and oxygen as a comparable amount of tissue in the rest of the body. The major part of these nutrients are used to keep the synaptic junctions working. It takes a lot of energy to think.

To operate at peak capacity the brain needs to be bathed in

oxygen and glucose. It also needs a steady supply of citric acid to facilitate the citric acid cycle and it needs sufficient supplies of simple elemental ions, especially calcium, potassium, and sodium. In upcoming chapters we will look at sources of choline and other nutrients for the brain. If there is a severe shortage of essential nutrients like citric acid or minerals, brain function is obviously impaired. If there is a long-term suboptimal level of these elements and nutrients, brain function suffers, but the deficit is difficult to detect.

Gamma-aminobutyric acid (GABA).   Another important neurotransmitter is gamma-aminobutyric acid (GABA). GABA is transmitted in much the same way as acetylcholine, by being stored in vesicles and released into the synaptic cleft when the signal arrives. The difference is that GABA inhibits the transmission of nerve signals.

It may seem strange that the nervous system would have end bulbs that inhibit the transmission of nerve impulses. Why not just have a system that efficiently sends the desired signals? As it turns out, such a plan doesn't work very well. Without inhibition neural networks rapidly become self-stimulating and run out of control quickly, sending signals faster and faster until the entire system is exhausted. The inhibitory endings prevent the firing of nerve cells from getting out of control. GABA is one of the most important inhibitory neurotransmitters.

Serotonin.   Serotonin is an inhibitory neurotransmitter that is probably controlled by a light-dark cycle. There is some experimental evidence that serotonin can produce sleep. Its precursor is tryptophan, which is converted into an intermediate product and then into serotonin, which is stored in the usual synaptic vesicles until its release is triggered. Bananas are a good source of tryptophan, and tryptophan can also be bought as a nutritional supplement in health food stores.

Serotonin is probably a neurohormone, meaning that it acts

THE NEURON 33

on the overall functioning and mood setting of the brain in contrast to transmitters like acetylcholine and GABA, which act quickly and influence the transmission of specific information. Sleepiness is not what we usually regard as a form of thinking, but it is apparently the result of brain processes and certainly affects whether we feel like thinking or carrying out other tasks.

Dopamine. Other neurotransmitters that act like neurohormones are dopamine, norepinephrine, and the endorphins. Dopamine plays a critical role in the control of movement. When the dopamine-producing center deep in the base of the brain begins to die and disappear, the result is Parkinson's disease. It is marked by a definite tremor and repetitive movements. L-dopa is a precursor of dopamine. When it is administered, the symptoms of Parkinsonism are reduced or eliminated.

Norepinephrine. Norepinephrine is secreted by a small group of cells in the brain stem that then connect with most areas of the brain. It seems to release this hormone, which has adrenaline-like effects on the capillaries of the brain and on some nerve cells. It probably increases blood flow to the brain and acts like amphetamine on the nerve cells to arouse brain activity. This hormone is also produced by the adrenal glands and acts as a stimulant in the body as well as in the brain. It is involved in the fight-or-flight reaction to danger.

Endorphins. The endorphins are neurohormones that are released in response to stress and to mark positive outcomes of behavior. Endorphins reduce the awareness of pain and irritation. They are natural painkillers. They are also released when behavior leads to a desire outcome. In this way these neurohormones act as a source of pleasure and reward.

The endorphins were found by scientists who were searching for natural parallels to morphine and other opiates. It seemed that there ought to be a natural form of these chemicals. The natural neurohormones have the same function of killing pain and giving pleasure that the opiates do. There is some evidence that drug addiction is triggered by low production of the endorphins. Addicts turn to drugs to make up for the felt lack of the natural neurohormones.

Lipofuscin. Lipofuscin is not a neurotransmitter, but it is a by-product of cell metabolism that is important when we consider the effects of brain aging. Lipofuscin (also called "age pigment") is cellular garbage. It accumulates mainly in brain cells and the skin. When these accumulations become visible on the skin, they are often called "liver spots." Lipofuscin deposits in brain cells inhibit and disrupt normal activity and can eventually cause the death of the cell. Some "smart pills" act to remove lipofuscin deposits, thus reversing a part of the aging process.

Studying the Function of the Brain

The brain is a remarkably difficult organ to study. The heart has yielded up its secrets rather easily, but we cannot say the same about the brain. We have seen how there is a good understanding of the functioning of the basic unit of the brain, the neuron. But we have a poor understanding of the larger action of the brain. We do not know exactly how memories are laid down or how the brain engages in thought.

We saw that the brain has one hundred billion neurons and that the center of action for those neurons is in the synapse. If we assume that there are an average of one thousand synapses for each cell, then the brain has in the neighborhood of one hundred trillion synaptic connections. These synapses are not the simple one-function connections we are accustomed to in modern electronic devices. Each synapse can carry a variety of messages and has very complex functions when large groups of neurons are acting as a neuronal net.

Beyond the Neuron

The brain is amazingly compact and complex. It is truly a mystery computer. Imagine that you were given a computer of such incredible complexity and small size that you were told to study. Also assume that this computer is as tightly packed with circuits as the brain—and as delicate. What would you do?

For one thing, you could put messages into the computer and see what it does in response. So you put in a simple problem in arithmetic like "What is 573 added to 382?" and the computer prints out an answer, "955." This tells you something about what it can do, but not much. And it tells you nearly nothing about what and how it operates. So you might give it more complicated instructions. We do the same thing with people and animals by giving tests and studying the results. A simple task like remembering numbers or a list of names and then writing them down later is a test of memory function.

Testing memory and reasoning skills with animals is more difficult because they cannot talk to us. Instead we construct mazes or have them press levers in response to cues such as sounds or colored lights. This is done for rewards and gives us some understanding of the capacities of the nervous system. We learn how much animals can learn and how long it takes them to form memories.

Another thing you might do with your mystery computer is to test it to see how it behaves when you alter the current level. It needs electricity to operate, and perhaps you might learn something by seeing how it works with a lower power input. Perhaps it will make more mistakes or give other indications about how it works.

We can do the same with people or animals by having them perform tasks with less food or by eliminating an essential nutrient from their diet. Often the first indication of a nutritional deficiency is in mental functioning. This gives us valuable information about the necessity of certain nutrients for good mental functioning as we shall see in the following chapters. Here we have an advantage over the study of a computer. A computer runs on electricity. The brains of humans and animals run on a variety of nutrients and oxygen. By reducing one or more of these essential nutrients, we can learn how the brain responds by testing behavior.

We might also increase the level of power to our computer to see if there is a change in functioning. The same can be done with humans and animals. Some nutrients make little or no difference when increased in amount. If you have a severe protein deficiency, you will have trouble thinking. Getting enough protein will enable you to think normally. But eating plenty of steak will not make you smarter. On the other hand, choline, one of the constituents of acetylcholine, may actually improve mental functioning. These effects are studied by altering the diet of volunteers or experimental animals.

Another way of studying the computer is to remove parts of it. We can easily see that this is a poor way of studying any delicate instrument. You really can't learn much about a computer with a hatchet and the same is true of a brain.

With animals, parts of the brain are removed to study the effects on learning and other tasks. With humans, injuries, strokes, and operations to correct problems like epilepsy serve as the source of such studies. In both cases, the results tell us something, but only on a very broad level. You do not get much detailed information from a damaged brain.

Another approach is to study the circuitry more directly. This gives much better information, but the ability to tease out patterns from something as compact and microscopic as the brain is extremely limited. We can follow some of the axons from one part of the brain to another, but there are such massive numbers of axons that a complete study is presently impossible. The situation is even more difficult for studying patterns of synaptic interconnection. At present the best knowledge has been gained about the visual information processes of the brain. We know how the brain picks out elements of an image like lines and curves, but we know almost nothing about what it does with that information.

Experiments in Understanding

In this book we will often refer to experiments with information processing and memory. Keep in mind that these experiments tell us something about how a person or animal is functioning mentally, but the experiment gives us a narrow window on overall functioning. Learning that a drug or nutrient enables a rat to learn a maze more quickly tells us something valuable about overall mental functioning. Maze learning does not exist in rats independently of other mental functions. If a human can memorize lists of words more easily with a drug such as Diapid (see Chapter 10), that ability to memorize probably extends to the ability to memorize many different kinds of information.

When you get information about experiments that measure the ability of rats to run through a maze or to choose the right lever, keep in mind that the measurement of these mental abilities can have great importance in understanding brain processes. There is not much difference between the functioning of the neurons in a rat's brain or in a human brain. The fundamental unit has remained largely unchanged during the course of mammalian evolution. What has changed is the pattern of development in different areas of the brain and the wealth of synaptic connections between areas.

By maximizing the health and functioning of the neuron, we maximize the basic building block of mental performance and intelligence. Nutrients have a strong influence in this process of optimizing mental functioning. Some recent breakthrough discoveries in drug research hold out the promise of increased mental functioning by improving the flow of oxygen to the brain, by improving the formation of memories, and by facilitating the flow of information through the brain.

Neurotransmitters are the "chemical messengers" that brain cells use to communicate with each other. The neurotransmitters controlling brain function and mental processes will receive special attention in this book. Several of the "smart pills" described in this book work by increasing the level of these neurotransmitters.

As our discussion unfolds, this information about brain structure and function will help clarify both how and why specific drugs and nutrients enhance intelligence and retard brain aging.

Enhancing intelligence is an immediate effect of the drugs and nutrients covered in this book. However, the power of these substances to maintain intelligence and prevent brain aging and senility is of greater long-term importance. Prevention is always better than cure, especially when given the painful emotional scars of senility. Nature does not play favorites. Individuals who incorporate good nutrition and health habits into their lifestyle will benefit the most.

3
Memory

It is said that, in old age, the memory is the first mental capacity to go. Actually, it is the first loss that we notice. It is difficult to be aware of being more or less creative for most people. We do not notice the gradual loss of the sense of smell or a decrease in reasoning power. But we do notice when we are unable to recall recent events or the name of someone we met last week.

There are clearly two sides to the coin of memory. We want to enhance it, and we want to avoid losing it in old age. Perhaps no other mental difficulty is as aggravating as trying to remember something and being unable to retrieve the memory despite the feeling that it is "on the tip of one's tongue."

We do not know how memory works, but we certainly rely on it. You depend on your ability to look up a telephone number and remember it long enough to dial your call. You park your car and expect to remember where it is hours later when you need it. You get to know someone well and expect to remember both the face and the name if you meet that individual years later. In each case we are frustrated or embarrassed if memory fails us.

Research shows that there are three kinds of memory, and certain nutrients and drugs can enhance each of the three kinds. The earliest discovery was the difference between short-term and long-term memory. Short-term memory enables us to remember a telephone number long enough to dial it. We can store about seven bits of information long enough to use it. That's why the telephone company chose to use seven digit numbers. Adding an area code usually is not a problem because it is usually associated with a city and remembered as a single unit.

After we use a telephone number frequently enough, we can remember it without effort. There has been a change and the number is stored in long-term memory. With short-term memory, we may have to repeat the number over and over to keep from losing it. If we are distracted, the number can easily be forgotten. But with long-term memory we make no effort to hold on to the number, and distractions do not cause us to forget it. We can go for days and weeks without using that number and still remember it when needed.

It is clear that some sort of change has taken place in the nervous system, but research has yet to establish exactly what kind of change has occurred. After looking at some of the important features of memory we will return to the question of what changes when we store something in long-term memory.

Besides short- and long-term memory, we also have working memory. This was discovered experimentally by an unfortunate operation performed in 1953 at a hospital in Connecticut. A young man, H.M., came in for treatment for severe seizures. He was desperate for a cure. At that time removal of the anterior portion of one temporal lobe was a standard surgical treatment for seizures that could not be helped with medication. This case was so severe that the doctors decided to remove parts of both temporal lobes.

The result was that both his seizures stopped but his ability to form new memories was lost. This came as a complete surprise to all involved. The key damage appears to have been to an area of the brain called the hippocampus and nearby structures. The hippocampus lies deep in the brain and is one of the oldest structures in evolutionary terms. It appears to be an important element in the brain's ability to form new memories.

H.M. did not lose his ability to recall events that happened before the operation. He could recognize old friends and discuss events that happened in the past. But if he met someone new and that person left the room briefly, he would be unable to recall having met that person. A momentary distraction was enough to break his awareness of whatever had just happened.

He could recall telephone numbers, but only by repeating them over and over to himself. Any distraction at all would immediately obliterate the memory of the number. So his short-term memory was operating, even though it was very faulty.

He could remember events that had happened before the operation, so his ability to recall long-term memories was not lost. But he seemed unable to form any new memories. One experiment showed that he could learn in a limited way. He was shown a simple puzzle consisting of a board with three posts on it. On one of the posts there were seven discs, each smaller than the one below it. The aim of the puzzle was to move the discs from one post to another one at a time without placing a larger disc on a smaller disc.

H.M. could understand the instructions and, with a great deal of effort, he was able to solve the puzzle. The next day he was shown the puzzle again. Of course, he had no memory of it, so it was explained to him again. This time it took a little less time to solve it. Finally after several learning sessions he was able to solve the puzzle quickly and easily. Each time he had no memory of having seen the puzzle before, and he expressed amazement that he was able to solve it so quickly.

This experiment shows the importance of working memory. This is the kind of memory that enables us to recall where the car is hours after we have parked it. With working memory we can store important information for a short period of time, recall it and then forget it, if necessary. The memory can also be passed on to long-term memory. For example, if you are new in a city, you might use your working memory to remember that you parked your car on Fifth Street near Market. After you drive off, you will probably forget where you parked you car that day, but you very well may form a permanent memory of the location where Fifth and Market intersect. It becomes part of the map you are forming of the city.

It seems that there is a period of time required for memories to shift from working to long-term memory. That seems to be about twenty minutes. One piece of evidence for this is the fact that people who are knocked unconscious and suffer a mild concussion often forget events that preceded the injury by twenty minutes or less. Sometimes longer periods of memory are obliterated. The blow interrupts the process by which the brain lays down permanent memories. It doesn't interfere with recall of memories that have already been formed, so the twenty-minute period for formation of long-term memories seems likely.

A related problem, Korsakoff's syndrome, is caused by alcoholism. It takes many years for the problem to appear. Like H.M., these patients have severe problems with memory. They are easily distracted from a short-term memory task and cannot recall anything that happened before they were distracted. They cannot remember the name or face of someone they just met if the person leaves the room for a few minutes. Postmortem examination of their brains shows that a relay area, the midline nuclei of the thalamus, is damaged, but the hippocampal area is relatively undamaged.

What we learn from these two types of memory disorders is that short-term memories pass into some sort of temporary holding pattern in the brain, and those memories that are important to us are then passed onto permanent storage. The areas such as the hippocampus and related structures participate in the formation of memories but do not store them. If the memories were stored there, all memory would be abolished, but H.M. could remember events that occurred before the operation.

How Memories Are Formed

There have been several theories advanced to account for how memories are laid down in the nervous system. The main element in any successful theory has to be identifying a change or changes in the structure of the neuron or in groups of neurons that can account for the permanent nature of long-term memory. Something in the brain has to change in order to preserve memory traces.

One theory was that the proteins in cells that carry information through the cell also stored the memories. This substance, messenger RNA, seemed like a good candidate, except for the problem of accounting for how it might control the flow of bioelectric currents through the cell. One piece of evidence in favor of this theory is that molecular activity in the neurons increases when experimental animals are learning new tasks.

The messenger RNA might be involved in changes in the cell structure, but it does not take part in the formation and transmission of bioelectric currents in the neuron. It is clearly the control of these currents that determines the action of the brain and nervous system on the inflow of sensory information, processing of that information, and transmitting action orders to the muscles. The messenger RNA theory has largely been discarded lately, although the RNA may be involved in guiding the changes in other areas of the cell that result in the formation of memories.

Another theory is that new synapses are formed to "hard wire" the circuits of memory. This depends on the notion that the brain is structured like a circuit board and forms new memories by introducing new circuits that alter the flow of information. There is solid evidence that the brain increases the number of synaptic connections when it is learning. Rats that were raised in "enriched" environments that gave them plenty of interesting objects to investigate developed brains that had many more synapses between axons and dendrites than rats that were raised in bare cages.

Unfortunately for this theory, there do not appear to be any identifiable patterns of synaptic growth that correspond to memory traces. Another problem is that it takes too long for new synapses to form. The crucial time for transferring memories from working to long-term memory (about twenty minutes) is too little time for the development of new circuits. Given the tremendous capacity for the human brain to form memories, our heads would have to be enormous to hold all our memories if the brain used this system for storing memories.

The most likely theory for memory formation comes from the study of a slimy sea creature, the sea hare or *Aplysia*. The sea hare is about six inches long, brown, and looks like a large garden slug. It has a nervous system that is quite simple and regular in structure. Each sea hare has a similar number and arrangement of nerve cells. But as simple as they are, they are capable of both short-term and long-term memory. Also they form these memories without growing complex patterns of new synaptic connections.

Eric Kandel is one of the scientists who have been working with these animals. He points out that there is little difference between the structure and function of neurons in humans, animals, and the sea hare.[1] The arrangement of the neurons into networks may be vastly different in each species, but the activity of the basic unit, the neuron, is fundamentally the same.

What he has discovered is that the behavior of the synaptic junction changes depending on the kind of incoming stimulation. The electrical signals that travel down the axon vary according to what the dendrites receive. What changes is the response at the end bulb. Different signals lead to changes in the amount of neurotransmitter released and even a change in the effect of the released transmitter substance on the receptor site. The details of this process are currently being investigated.

Another feature of the behavior of the synaptic junction is that it can change in response to more than one new stimulus at a time. What appears to happen is that networks of neurons act as a gang in response to different inputs. This means that memory is stored in diffuse areas of the brain, and the same neural networks can form many new memories at the same time. This avoids the cumbersome problem of forming specific circuits for each individual memory.

This theory of synaptic alteration also accounts for the fact that memories appear to be stored throughout the cerebral cortex. If part of the brain is cut out, specific memories are not lost. Instead the memory traces that remain are less clear. It is like taking a photograph and making it more fuzzy. The images remain, but they are harder to recognize clearly.

The synaptic alteration theory has direct implications for the effect of nutrients and drugs on memory. By increasing the availability of acetylcholine, oxygen, and other metabolites, the synaptic end bulb may be better able to produce the changes that lead to memory formation. Some of the experimental evidence that will be reviewed in the following chapters lends support to this possibility.

Another important implication of this synaptic alteration theory is that the loss of memory associated with Alzheimer's disease and other degenerative changes in the brain are the result of synaptic destruction. The illustrations of degenerated neurons show that the worst effects are on the wealth of synaptic connections. Optimal nourishment of the synaptic junction and protecting it from damage are of paramount importance if we are to enhance our memory and preserve it.

4

Free Radicals and Antioxidants

Physical aging and mental deterioration are emerging as one of America's major health problems as the average age of the population continues to rise. What is the source of the loss of intelligence and health that we associate with aging? Why do some people remain clear of mind and sound of body well into their eighties, nineties, and beyond? Is it possible to avoid the debility of old age and even to increase our mental powers?

The Free Radical Theory of Aging

The answer to these questions may come from the research of Dr. Denham Harman at the University of Nebraska. He has developed the free radical theory of aging, which explains the physical and mental deterioration that usually accompanies chronological aging.[1] His discovery is as revolutionary and profound in its implications for medicine and the treatment of chronic degenerative diseases as was the germ theory and the development of antibiotics for the treatment of infectious diseases.

Dr. Harman found that our bodies are being attacked constantly by what scientists call "free radicals." In simple terms, a free radical is a molecule with a free or unpaired electron. Chemical compounds are most stable when electrons exist in pairs. A free radical with its unpaired electron is highly unstable and extremely dangerous.

Another way of understanding the power of a free radical is to say that a free radical is a molecule that lacks an electron. A free radical is extremely reactive because it is electrochemically unbalanced. It will steal an electron from another molecule, and thus regain its stability by again becoming an electron pair. It gets the electron it needs by violently tearing it away from another molecule. The molecule that is attacked by a free radical is damaged and often destroyed. The accumulation of free radical damage leads to the chronic degenerative diseases that are associated with aging.[2]

Free radicals are neutralized by substances in the body called "antioxidants". An antioxidant combines with a free radical to eliminate the destructive power of the extra electron.

Shortly we will learn more about free radicals and antioxidants. But for now we can make the following statement based on Dr. Harman's research: Free radicals are killers and antioxidants may be life savers!

Aging and Chronic Degenerative Disease

Aging is the number one health problem today in developed countries.[3] Chronic degenerative diseases are merely the visible symptoms of unhealthy life styles. Aging should be a natural process, free of illness, and without serious loss of mental or physical abilities. Instead, chronic degenerative diseases are an epidemic, crippling the citizens of industrial nations as they age.

Chronic degenerative diseases are more commonly known by their individual names: strokes, arthritis, heart disease, arteriosclerosis, senility, cancer, etc. The insidious damage these diseases produce is obvious. But the underlying cause of these diseases is found at the cellular level—the actual destruction of cells.[4]

The "agents of destruction" are the free radicals that are gradually destroying cells in the body.

The Chain Reaction

When a free radical steals an electron away from another molecule, it creates new free radicals. The newly generated free radicals each create more, and a self-propagating chain reaction results. One unchecked free radical does not produce just one damaging hit. The chain reaction it creates can multiply its damaging effects a million times or more.[5]

You may be able to understand the effects of a free radical chain reaction by visualizing the following scene.

Imagine that you are sitting in the bleachers of a gymnasium. Create an empty basketball court in your mind's eye. There are no people present, but as you look closer, you see that the entire floor is covered with mouse traps, sitting neatly side by side, row after row. It takes almost two hundred thousand mouse traps to fill a regulation basketball court. Looking closer, you see that each mouse trap is set in its cocked position, ready to spring and, on the snapping arm of each mouse trap, rests a single Ping-Pong ball.

The scene is quiet and undisturbed. Now, there is an extra Ping-Pong ball that represents a single free radical sitting on the bleacher next to you. You take the Ping-Pong ball, stand up and throw it far out onto the floor. You can "see" what is going to happen.

The Ping-Pong ball is going to start a chain reaction and within seconds, hundreds of thousands of mouse traps and Ping-Pong balls are being set off. Each flying Ping-Pong ball represents a free radical generated by the chain reaction, and each flying Ping-Pong ball is capable of starting its own free radical chain reaction. This demonstrates how a single free radical can initiate a chain reaction of destruction, producing massive damage in our body's cells.

Excess free radicals produce a cascade of chain reactions, multiplying their damage by a million times or more. In fact, one of the best ways scientists have to investigate this phenomenon is by studying the trail of damage molecules and cells left in the wake of uncontrolled free radical reactions. This destruction and loss of cells is the cause of the aging process.

Damage to Genetic Messages

Every day of our lives, old cells die and new ones are produced. DNA molecules carry the genetic code that tells the new cells how to function. Another kind of molecule, RNA, carries the messages through the cell and directs cellular activity. DNA and RNA are especially susceptible to free radical damage.[6]

You can understand this damage to DNA and RNA by carrying out another visualization experiment. Imagine a huge, bright theater marquee with thousands of bulbs. The flashing bulbs create a message that is easy to read. When a few bulbs are burned out, the message is still clear. However, as time passes, more and more bulbs burn out. Soon it becomes difficult, and finally impossible to make out the intended message.

When free radical damage causes "more and more of the lights to go out" on DNA and RNA molecules, the body's directions on how to repair and make new cells become less and less clear. New cells are unable to perform properly, and eventually some of them may become cancerous. The result of this cumulative damage to the genetic blueprint is chronic degenerative disease and death.

Sources of Free Radicals

Free radicals come from sources both inside and outside the body. Internally, free radicals are produced during the body's own metabolic activities. With optimal nutrition, the body neutralizes most of the free radicals that are normally produced.

The white blood cells of the immune system are potent generators of free radicals, using them as a means of destroying disease-causing organisms. Some of the external or environmental sources of free radical exposure are sunlight and other sources of ultraviolet light, X rays, chemical toxins in our air, water and food, peroxidized fats, and nuclear radiation.

The two most harmful sources of free radical exposure to humans in terms of the amount of damage relative to the frequency of exposure are cigarette smoking and rancid fats.

Cigarette smoking generates enormous quantities of free radicals. The high temperature at the burning tip of a cigarette provides the energy needed to knock off millions of electrons, creating free radicals, which are inhaled in the smoke. The tars in the smoke are also potent chemicals that generate free radicals.

Fats and oils (chemically referred to as lipids) are a major source of free radicals. Most of the lipids in our bodies come from fats in the foods we eat. The free radical theory gives us a new perspective on fats in our diet. Oxygen reacts with unsaturated fats to produce free radicals as the fat or oil becomes rancid and spoils. These free radicals in turn react with the rest of the fat or oil, creating a free radical chain reaction of destruction. Many scientists now believe that the oxidation of unsaturated fats is the primary cause of aging in the human cell.[7] Because the brain contains the highest percentage of unsaturated fats of any part of the body, free radicals can do more damage to that organ. This makes it especially important to consume a high level of antioxidants to prevent damage and aging of brain cells.

How Fats Are Oxidized or Spoiled

Exposure to air (oxygen) and heat are two factors that greatly increase the oxidation of fats and consequently, the production of free radicals. Thus, cooking creates ideal conditions for the oxidation of fats. The higher the temperature and the longer the cooking process, the greater the degree of oxidation and free radical production.

The cooking of meat is a good example. The best cuts ·of meat may contain as much as 60 percent fat. This is now recognized as one of the major reasons why meat-eating societies have a much higher incidence of heart disease.

When you eat french fries and fried chicken, you are eating food cooked in oil at high temperatures. This food has been soaked in free radical-generating oxidized fat.

Fast-food establishments are the worst offenders in this area. They turn their deep-fat fryers on in the morning and the oils are kept at a high temperature and exposed to air all day long. How often do they change the oil in the deep fryer? Changing the oil is like throwing money down the drain to the manager or owner who has to buy the oil.

Partially hydrogenated fats also contribute to cellular degeneration and aging. The process of partial hydrogenation was developed by the food processing industry for two reasons. First, it enabled them to turn liquid oils into semisolid fat to gain the desired consistency for commercial products. Second, the process extends the shelf life of the oils. However, hydrogenation removes important nutrients and alters the structure of fats. These altered fats are toxic to your body. See Chapter 27 for a complete discussion of fats and oils.

Antioxidants

Pollution, stress, and toxic additives in food cause cellular damage. It is almost impossible to avoid these things in our industrialized world. However, we can prevent much of the damage by the proper use of compounds called antioxidants.

Antioxidants are substances that have the ability to protect the body's cells against the chemical reactions that form free radicals. The human cell uses essential enzymes and nutrients to maintain the body's protective antioxidant system. This system is supposed to prevent the uncontrolled free radical chain reactions that cause age-related diseases.

Some of the most important enzymes and nutrients required for maintaining the protective antioxidant system are:

Vitamins:	vitamin C (ascorbic acid), vitamin E vitamin B-2 (riboflavin), vitamin B-3 (niacinamide), and vitamin A (or beta-carotene)
Minerals:	selenium, zinc, copper, iron, manganese
Amino acids:	L-cysteine, L-methionine
Enzymes:	glutathione peroxidase, superoxide dismutase

Where do these protective antioxidants come from? The enzymes are manufactured in the body. The other items are obtained from the diet or from nutritional supplements. We will cover the major antioxidant nutrients (beta-carotene, vitamins A, E, C, and the mineral selenium) in individual chapters.

Antioxidant Enzymes

Antioxidant enzymes are manufactured by the body for one purpose only . . . to protect you. Two antioxidant enzymes important to health and the aging process are superoxide dismutase and glutathione peroxidase.

Superoxide Dismutase/SOD

Oxygen is a double-edged sword. We need oxygen for life, but oxygen-free radicals produced in the body can be killers. Superoxide dismutase is an antioxidant enzyme that has the job of protecting us against the damage from oxygen free radicals. Our bodies produce energy by burning food with oxygen. This is called metabolism. During these metabolic processes, many oxygen free radicals are generated.

One of the most common free radicals is called the superoxide free radical or the superoxide radical. It is the job of the superoxide dismutase enzyme to neutralize the superoxide radicals before they are able to start any free radical chain reaction.

The superoxide dismutase enzyme deactivates the highly reactive, poisonous superoxide free radical, converting it to hydrogen peroxide and oxygen. Hydrogen peroxide is also a free radical, but it is much less reactive than the superoxide free radical. An enzyme called catalase then breaks down hydrogen peroxide to oxygen and water. Antioxidants, like SOD, react with free radicals to deactivate them. This keeps the free radicals from attacking cells, thereby preventing cell damage and biological aging.

There are two types of SOD; one exists inside the mitochondria and the other exists inside the cell, but outside the mitochondria. The form of SOD found inside the mitochondria has the mineral manganese as its central element. The other form of SOD has the minerals zinc and copper in its structure. Research has shown that marginal dietary deficiencies of any of these three minerals can produce a reduction in SOD activity. Reduced SOD activity exposes an individual to increased levels of superoxide free radical-induced cellular damage and biological aging.

Therapeutic Benefits of SOD

Some of the reported benefits associated with superoxide dismutase are quite remarkable. It has been shown that SOD can help to protect against and heal arthritis, help to protect against cancer, and help to retard the aging process. Research has shown that SOD has potential as a therapeutic agent, but not in the oral forms that are being sold as nutritional supplements. Tests show that SOD taken orally is not effective. The enzyme is destroyed by stomach acids and digestive enzymes. The SOD enzyme is such a large molecule that if any did get through the stomach, it could not be absorbed through the intestinal wall. The injectable form of SOD has been used in the above research but this form of SOD is not available as a commercial product. It is, however, an approved veterinary drug.

It appears that we are faced with a dilemma. Superoxide dismutase is an important antioxidant, antiaging enzyme, but it is not effective when taken orally. Is there an answer?

Make Your Own SOD

When you supply your body with optimal levels of nutrition, your body will make its own SOD. Zinc, copper, and manganese are the essential minerals needed for the biosynthesis of SOD enzymes. Individuals whose diets are marginally deficient in these minerals are known to have significantly reduced SOD enzyme activity. Good diet and nutritional supplements are the best way to insure maximum SOD enzyme activity in your body.

Glutathione Peroxidase

Glutathione peroxidase is another important antioxidant enzyme produced in the body. This enzyme is receiving a lot of attention because of the many different ways it acts to protect our systems. Glutathione peroxidase:

1. Is a strong antioxidant.
2. Helps protect against alcohol-induced liver damage.
3. Reactivates vitamin C, which then reactivates vitamin E.
4. Combines with toxic metals to eliminate them from the body.
5. Improves the immune system's ability to destroy bacteria.
6. Shows promise as a cancer preventive agent because it can destroy cancer-causing substances such as epoxides and peroxides.

The glutathione peroxidase enzyme has a number of components. Each molecule of the enzyme contains four atoms of the mineral, selenium. Another component is glutathione, which is made up of the amino acids cysteine, glutamic acid, and glycine. We need these three amino acids and selenium to keep this protective enzyme system functioning.

It has recently been discovered that the component, glutathione, is absorbed well when taken orally. Glutathione supplements are also available in most health food stores. However, what is really important is that your diet supplies your body with all the nutrients it needs to produce the complete enzyme, glutathione peroxidase.

Final Comments

The free radical theory of aging is gaining wide acceptance. Basically, it states that increased exposure to free radicals and free radical–generating agents causes aging and chronic degenerative diseases. Antioxidant nutrients protect the body against free radical damage. Higher levels of antioxidants in your body will protect against the development of chronic degenerative disease and will contribute to both a longer and a healthier life. These advances in our understanding of the biochemistry of health are enabling us to make the first real progress in the areas of life extension, reversing the aging process and enhancing intelligence.

II

IMPROVING
PERFORMANCE

5

Introduction to Improving Mental Performance

Over the years records in all sports continue to be broken, and the level of human athletic performance continues to improve. We do not know what or where the limits lie or when they will be reached. I would like to suggest that a similar condition and situation is possible with the human mind. Is it not possible, even logical and probable, that we can find ways to improve and increase the performance of our minds? Good nutrition combined with exercise leads to improved athletic performance. By lifting weights we can become stronger and lift more weight.

What about nourishing, training, and flexing our mental muscles? Can it be done? Research shows that it is indeed possible, but we need to make the same level of commitment to intellectual excellence as does the champion athlete to physical performance.

We do not yet know what optimum levels of intelligence are, but research is showing us the way to increase intelligence and mental capabilities. I am not suggesting that we can go beyond either maximum athletic performances or similar maximum intellectual capabilities. What I am saying is that since very few people even approach their maximum capabilities, we need to maximize the potential that we do have.

Ways of Improving Performance

If we want to improve our mental capacities, just what do we need to do to accomplish this? Exercise and proper diet are the foundation in both improving and maintaining high levels of both physical and mental performance. However, this section will focus primarily on cognitive enhancers, herbal preparations and nutrients that are capable of enhancing memory, learning, recall, and other mental functions.

There are a number of ways that substances can act to improve cognitive functions. They can:

1. Increase the level of neurotransmitters in the brain.
2. Improve brain cell metabolism.
3. Optimize the action of certain enzymes.
4. Increase the supply of oxygen to brain cells.
5. Dissolve and remove cellular garbage deposits from cells.
6. Improve the level of electrical activity in the brain.

Advances in modern technology are responsible for the sudden emergence of this new area, cognitive enhancement. For example, the new high-powered electron microscopes enable us to see smaller, look deeper, and understand more than we ever have. Until recently, we could only look at brain cells. Now we can actually look inside brain cells. We are now able to look at both the structures and the processes of the brain and learn how they function. This is giving us clues on ways to enhance information processing capabilities and improve the brain's memory, storage, and retrieval processes.

6

Intelligence, Thinking, and Learning

What is intelligence? Scientists from the disciplines of psychology, physiology, genetics, biochemistry, and neuroanatomy have been seeking the answer to this question for years. To date, there is still no comprehensive definition of intelligence. Perhaps we cannot accurately define intelligence, but we can certainly tell when it is missing.

In the attempt to understand intelligence, we seek to find ways to measure it. Not all of these approaches are useful. Professor Edwin Boring of Harvard, writing in *The New Republic* in 1923 said, "Intelligence as a measurable capacity must at the start be defined as the capacity to do well in an intelligence test. Intelligence is what the tests test."[1] This is no doubt true once we agree on a test, but how do we arrive at agreement on the test that will define intelligence for us?

It becomes a matter of defining the concept of intelligence before we really understand what it is. For example, a test that excluded measurements of verbal ability or logical thinking would not be considered an intelligence test. But what about measuring relationship skills, manual dexterity, or the ability to create art or music? We make a subjective judgment when we decide what to include or eliminate in setting up the test.[2]

Scientists still disagree about what should be measured when studying intelligence, the methods of measurement, and the interpretation of the results. Many authorities agree that there are many kinds of intelligence, and that current intelligence tests only measure part of our human capabilities.

Why is it that the brain and what it can do is so difficult to understand? One part of the answer has to do with the complexity of the brain. Sitting on top of our shoulders is a three-pound gray, wrinkled mass that is estimated to contain between 10 and 15 *billion* nerve cells, which are capable of making 10 to the 800th power connections![3] Numbers this large are literally beyond the comprehension of the human mind. Also inside our brains are somewhere between 100,000 and 1,000,000 different chemicals at work. Our brains are incredibly complex.

To further complicate matters, there is the problem of getting inside the brain to watch it work. The working parts are extremely small and most people who are alive are reluctant to volunteer their brains for this kind of research. As a result, we have to work with animals.

Scientists realize that we are in the infancy of our understanding of the brain. However, what we learn in the future about the capabilities of our brains will determine the future of mankind. I believe that the mind is the next frontier, and that it will prove to be the most exciting frontier mankind has ever explored.

The Myth of a Fixed Intelligence

Is our intelligence determined at birth by our genetic makeup or can it be developed in response to our environment? This is one of the oldest debates about intelligence—the issue of Nature vs. Nurture. I believe that both our genetic inheritance and our environment are involved in the outcome.

There is an ever increasing volume of research that indicates that mental functioning can be improved. Intelligence, memory, and learning respond to many factors. The research documented in this book has reported many aspects of diet, nutrition, and life style that support this. These influences that improve intelligence are classified as environmental factors (as opposed to genetic factors).

There is some fascinating research that has taken a quantum leap in breaking down the old idea of a fixed intelligence. The pioneering research of the neuroanatomist Dr. Marian Diamond, and her co-workers at the University of California at Berkeley, shows that intelligence, the ability to learn, and even the physical brain itself can be developed. She has recently reported the story of this work in her book, *Enriching Heredity: The Impact of the Environment on the Anatomy of the Brain.*[4]

The Diamond group has been studying how the brains of rats change in response to different environments. The rat brain resembles the human brain in many aspects of both form and functioning. The researchers created three different environmental test conditions: the impoverished environment, the normal environment, and the enriched environment.

In the impoverished environment, a single rat would be left alone in a regular-sized laboratory cage. The normal environment consisted of three rats in a regular-sized laboratory cage. The enriched environment was a larger-sized cage with twelve rats and numerous toys.

Every few days the rats were taken out of the cages for a few minutes to clean the cages. In the enriched environment, the toys would be randomly placed back in the cage before returning the rats to the cage. The rats in this environment would scurry around, examining and exploring the toys and their new placement.

The results of these experiments show that access to stimulating objects and a stimulating environment produces a thicker cerebral cortex—a bigger brain! The researchers found that the enriched environment produced both more brain cells and larger brain cells! Other researchers have shown that these conditions facilitate faster and more accurate problem solving, which is a key component of intelligence.[5]

Part of Diamond's research has shown that an impoverished

environment will inhibit brain growth, resulting in a decrease in the size and number of brain cells. This research has also shown that an enriched environment can overcome some of the negative aspects of stress and dietary protein deficiency experienced early in life.

Diet, nutrition, the air we breathe, and a stimulating environment can increase levels of important brain chemicals, producing bigger brain cells and faster learning. The brain can and does change in response to its environment.

Genetic inheritance is not destiny. Marian Diamond's research has shown that the brain, *at any stage of life*, from prenatal to old age, can increase in size and learn faster. Although she has used rats in her research, I feel that her work is making important statements about the potential of developing the human brain.

The results from these studies as well as the studies on the nutrients, drugs, and herbs reported in this book argue that our brains can continue to grow throughout our lives. We can truly expand our minds and our potential.

Thinking and Learning

Not only is there a need to maximize the conditions that will enable optimum development of intelligence and mental capabilities, there is also a great need to teach people how to think, to learn, and to reason. I believe that these skills can and should be taught.

It has been my experience that the traditional approach to education is not focused on developing effective methods to teach these skills. Instead, the emphasis is on learning facts and memorization.

A Gallup poll asked parents what they would most like their children to gain from their education. Most parents wanted their children "to learn how to think."[6]

I believe our minds are as instinctively motivated to learn as our legs are to walk. Just as the legs of a champion have to be trained, so our minds have to be taught and trained to function at their best.

Scientists from such diverse disciplines as neurophysiology and anthropology are finding evidence that the human brain changes in accordance with changes in understanding and awareness. In other words, as our understanding and awareness changes, the brain that has processed new information also changes. The more we know, the more we can know. The more we understand, the more we can understand. Learning how to think creates changes in the brain at the cellular level that facilitate better thinking.

Albert Einstein said,

> It is not so very important for a person to learn facts. For that he does not really need a college. He can learn them from books. The value of an education in a liberal arts college is not the learning of many facts but the training of the mind to think—something that cannot be learned from books.[7]

The art of thinking begins with a change in the individual's belief system about one's ability to think and about the nature of intelligence. It is true that we have much to learn about how the mind functions, but the first step is to acknowledge and understand what science has already proven—that our minds can grow and change. The research on intelligence, memory, learning, and the brain in this book leads to the conclusion that the critical issue is not whether it is possible to enhance intelligence and mental facilities, but how far we can go in enlarging the frontiers of the mind.

In addition to teaching the skill of thinking and learning, we also need to change the common attitude that answers are only right or wrong. In his book *Mindstorms*, Seymore Papert made the following comments about an attitude toward learning that is developed by many computer programers. He said,

Many children are held back in their learning because they have a model of learning in which you have either "got it" or "got it wrong." But when you program a computer you almost never get it right the first time. Learning to be a master programmer is learning to become highly skilled at isolating and correcting "bugs," the parts that keep the program from working. The question to ask about the program is not whether it is right or wrong, but if it is fixable. If this way of looking at intellectual products were generalized to how the larger culture thinks about knowledge and its acquisition, we all might be less intimidated by our fears about "being wrong."[8]

Children learning programming skills in grade school are developing a priceless by-product. They are developing a new attitude about errors and a new attitude and confidence about thinking and learning. When children have the will to stick with a problem and to examine and adjust their thinking until they can get something to work (on a computer or in life), an important level of confidence begins to grow. Discipline switches from an external and oppressing "get it right the first time" to an internal and intellectual "make it work."[9]

Buckminster Fuller was one of the outstanding minds of all time. In a speech about what the world would be like in the year 2000, he said, "The world's greatest resources are to be found in human intelligence, ingenuity, and imagination." Early in his life, Bucky discovered the secret of having a passion for learning and understanding life, and he spent the rest of his life trying to give that secret away to others.

In an editorial eulogizing Buckminster Fuller, Norman Cousins wrote the following,

If we read Bucky Fuller solely for information we will obtain information, but we will be cheating ourselves. We should read him for the increased respect he gives us for human potential, and for the lesson that there are no boundaries to the human mind, which he celebrates above all else.[10]

We can make Buckminster Fuller's dream a reality. There are no boundaries to the human mind.

7

Choline/Lecithin: A Vital Role in Memory

Choline and lecithin are important to mental functioning because they are precursors to acetylcholine, the most important neurotransmitter involved in memory and mental functioning. Without enough acetylcholine the brain cannot store memories or function properly.

Choline and lecithin are nutritional supplements that are available without a prescription. Choline seldom occurs by itself, being found most commonly as part of the lecithin molecule. Choline is actually classified as a member of the B vitamin group and is the precursor to acetylcholine.

Lecithin has several functions in the body:

1. Aids in the transportation of fats to the cells.
2. Helps to keep cholesterol soluble.
3. Increases the production of bile acids that are made from cholesterol.

By means of these three processes, lecithin helps to lower cholesterol levels, thus decreasing the risk of hardening of the arteries and heart disease.

Unfortunately the term "lecithin" has two meanings. This can lead to confusion on the part of consumers. By clarifying the meanings we can make better use of this important nutrient. First, in the health food industry and the scientific community the word "lecithin" is used to refer to phosphatidyl choline.

Second, to the food-processing industry, lecithin is the common name for a naturally occurring mixture of compounds called phospholipids, only a small percentage of which is phosphatidyl choline.

In this book, the commercial mixture will be referred to as "commercial lecithin" and the specific compound, phosphatidyl choline, will be called simply "lecithin."

Phosphatidyl choline is important to our discussion of intelligence and memory enhancement because:

1. It is a major structural component of brain cells.
2. The brain is able to use choline derived from phosphatidyl choline to make acetylcholine.

Since acetylcholine is the major chemical messenger for thoughts and memories, it is extremely important in the normal functioning of the brain as well as in any attempt to improve mental functioning.

Commercial lecithin is used by the food processing industry as an emulsifier. Commercial lecithin allows fat-soluble and water-soluble substances to mix, which gives food a pleasing consistency and texture.

Effects

Lecithin functions as a source of structural material for every cell in the human body, particularly those of the brain and nerves. In a healthy person, lecithin accounts for approximately 30 percent of the dry weight of the brain.[1] It aids in the metabolism of fats, regulates blood cholesterol, nourishes the fat-like sheaths of nerve fibers, and is a precursor to acetylcholine.

Choline and lecithin have been used with some success in treating Huntington's disease, tardive dyskinesia, Parkinson's disease, and other diseases of the nervous system.[2] All of these conditions produce an uncontrollable shaking and twitching that is sometimes seen in elderly people. Choline and lecithin are also used therapeutically to treat diabetes, gall bladder problems, liver disorders, muscular dystrophy, glaucoma, arterio-sclerosis, senility, and memory problems.

Choline for Infants

Newborn children have extremely high choline levels in their blood. This seems to be necessary for the manufacture of myelin, which is the material that insulates and protects the nervous system. Choline is also used in the synthesis of cell membranes within the brain and nervous system.

Human breast milk contains a much higher percentage of lecithin than cow's milk. Mother's milk may be extremely important in supplying adequate levels of choline for an infant's developing nervous system. Breast feeding is just the beginning of a lifetime of good nutrition.

Choline and Memory

For the brain to store a memory there has to be some kind of change at the cellular level. Permanent memories are laid down in the brain through changes in the way messages are transmitted between brain cells. The messages are sent from one brain cell to another by chemical messengers or neurotransmitters. Acetylcholine is the most important neurotransmitter involved with memory and thought transmission.

As we age, a number of changes occur that lead to memory loss. There can be a decrease in the activity of the enzyme that produces acetylcholine. Sometimes there is an increase in the activity of acetylcholinesterase, which is the enzyme that breaks down acetylcholine.

There can also be a decrease in receptor sites and/or a decrease in the receptor site's ability to "read" the message from the chemical messenger. Another problem is the actual free radical damage and destruction of the sensitive fatty structure of the brain cell dendrites themselves.

The bottom line is that as we age the brain tends to make less acetylcholine, more is destroyed, and thought and memory begin to suffer. We need to consume more of the sources of choline to make up for the deficit in the neurotransmitter, acetylcholine.

Enhancing Memory

Choline is able to pass through the blood-brain barrier where the brain utilizes it to make acetylcholine. Thus, choline enhances memory by increasing the amount of acetylcholine available for memory and thought processes.

A study of ten normal, healthy volunteers established the effect of a single oral dose of choline on two kinds of memory. One was a test of short-term memory. The other was a test that measured the ability to remember concrete words like "table" versus abstract words like "truth." The subjects were tested with either choline or a placebo.[3]

The test found an increase in short-term memory when members of the group were tested with choline. In addition, the memory of abstract words was improved. But the memory of concrete words was unaffected, probably because the initial rate of retention of concrete words was higher since concrete words are easier to remember. But the test did show that choline selectively enhanced the short-term recall of abstract words.

Food Sources

Food contains only trace amounts of free choline. Most of the choline normally present in our diet is in the form of lecithin. It occurs in most seed oils and in unrefined foods containing oil. The most common and best commercial source of lecithin is soybean oil, which contains up to 2 percent lecithin. The lecithin in soybean oil contains both essential fatty acids (57 percent Omega-6 and 9 percent Omega-3), whereas the lecithin from most other oils contains only Omega-6.[4]

The food processing industry is trying to develop genetic

OMEGA
3+6

strains of soybeans that will cut the Omega-3 content from 9 percent down to only 3 percent because Omega-3 spoils more quickly. Again, for longer shelf life and economic reasons, we sacrifice nutritional quality and compromise our health. The frightening thing is that the consumer is not aware of these changes or of their long-term consequences.

Other foods that are high in choline and lecithin are soybeans, egg yolks, liver, brewer's yeast, peanuts, peas, and beans. Other lesser sources are green leafy vegetables, cauliflower, cabbage, and cheese.

Supplements

Choline and lecithin are available as nutritional supplements and can be found at most health food stores. Pharmacies and other retail stores that carry vitamins are also possible sources.

Choline tablets and capsules are available commercially as the bitartrate salt, choline bitartrate. Choline is available in liquid form as the chloride salt, choline chloride.

Lecithin is available as granules, liquid, capsules, chewable tablets, or powder. For a long time, commercial lecithin had such a small percentage (about 5 percent) of the active ingredient phosphatidyl choline, it was almost worthless for memory improvement. Dosages had to be so large to be effective that few people were able to keep up a regular long-term dosage schedule.

Most of the research on the memory-enhancing capabilities of choline and lecithin has been published in the last several years. The health food industry has responded to this new information by producing and marketing commercial lecithin that contains higher percentages of the active ingredient, phosphatidyl choline. For therapeutic success, commercial lecithin should be at least 30 percent phosphatidyl choline. Read labels when buying lecithin to insure getting one of the newer products with higher phosphatidyl choline content. One of the newest products, called PC-55, contains 55 percent phosphatidyl choline.

Now that higher quality commercial lecithin products are available, the question as to whether to take choline or lecithin, is a toss-up. Some therapists and researchers prefer choline while others like lecithin. Since there is no overwhelming evidence favoring either product, it probably comes down to the personal preference of the therapist and the individual being treated.

Dosage Range

Choline must be given four times a day at doses of 2.5 to 3 grams per dose to keep blood levels of choline in the therapeutic range, whereas lecithin functions as a time-released form of choline and only needs to be taken twice daily.

Vitamin B-5 (pantothenic acid or calcium pantothenate) should be taken along with choline/lecithin because the brain requires ample vitamin B-5 to convert choline to acetylcholine. Vitamin B-5 is part of the enzyme that controls the choline to acetylcholine conversion.

Many studies have examined whether choline or lecithin can improve performance in memory and learning tasks. The results from these studies are not consistent. For example, some attempts to improve memory performance in extremely old humans and animals who have suffered considerable neurological deterioration have not had good results.

One reason for this inconsistency may be that the aged brain is unable to convert extra amounts of choline into acetylcholine. Also it may be necessary to improve other factors in aged brains before substantial therapeutic responses can be obtained, such as ensuring that adequate levels of vitamin B-5 are available.

Another possible explanation for these inconsistent results is that some research designs used low dosage levels. The blood levels of choline produced in these studies may not have been high enough to achieve therapeutic effects.

Deficiency Symptoms

A deficiency of choline can be associated with high cholesterol levels, some types of cardiac symptoms, skin problems such as psoriasis, poor tolerance of dietary fats, gastric ulcers, high blood pressure, gall stones, and liver disease.[5]

Choline/Lecithin Robbers

Alcohol, refined sugar, and refined flour deplete choline from the body. Lecithin occurs naturally in unrefined foods that contain oil. However, the major oil and food processing companies frequently remove lecithin in the process of "making food" because it can hasten spoilage.

Side Effects and Toxicity

CHOLINE CHLORIDE NO DIAREA

Choline therapy can produce two side effects that users should be aware of. An unpleasant aspect of high-dosage pure choline therapy is the development of a fishy odor. A large part of orally ingested choline is rapidly broken down by bacteria in the intestines. When this happens, a portion of the choline molecule called trimethylamine is liberated and this compound gives the body a fishy odor.[6]

Consumption of large doses of choline sometimes causes diarrhea. Starting at lower dosages and gradually building up to higher levels will help to avoid this.

Lecithin is metabolized differently than choline. It does not produce the fishy odor, nor does it produce the diarrhea that is common with choline therapy.

Contraindications

Compounds that act as precursors to acetylcholine such as choline, lecithin, and DMAE should not be used in patients who are manic depressive (DMAE will be discussed in the next chapter). Specifically, higher levels of acetylcholine can cause the depressive phase of a manic-depressive psychosis to deepen.[7]

Final Comments

Recently researchers have used the strategy of combining drugs in an effort to improve their memory-enhancing effects. Early reports from this frontier are very exciting. The degree of improvement can be far greater than the added effects of the individual drugs; the effect seems to be multiplied.

The drug combination study that "broke loose" this exciting and promising new area of investigation involves the use of choline in combination with piracetam.

8

DMAE/Deanol:
The Brain Stimulant

During the past few years DMAE, also known as deanol, has become well-known for its properties as a safe, natural brain stimulant. It appears to alter the levels of acetylcholine, an important neurotransmitter. Acetylcholine is involved in memory formation as well as thought processes. Results from the use of DMAE have shown that it elevates mood, improves memory and learning, increases intelligence, and extends lifespan.

The generic name for the drug discussed in this chapter is deanol. A generic name is a "common name" that is not protected by trademark registration. The chemical name for deanol is 2-dimethylaminoethanol. DMAE comes from the first letter of each syllable in the chemical name **Di-Methyl-Amino-Ethanol**.

Deanol and DMAE are used somewhat interchangeably in scientific literature. DMAE is the term that is used most commonly in nutritional catalogs and throughout the health food industry, and it is the term that will be used in this book.

Effects

DMAE is a naturally occurring nutrient that is found most abundantly in such "brain" foods as anchovies and sardines. Small amounts of DMAE occur naturally in the brain.[1] DMAE stimulates the production of choline, which in turn allows the brain to optimize production of acetylcholine. Acetylcholine is the primary neurotransmitter involved in learning and memory.

Deanol used to be marketed as a prescription drug by Riker Laboratories under the trade name Deaner. The FDA originally authorized Riker to market DMAE and label it as "possibly effective" for the following indications:

1. Learning problems associated with underachieving and shortened attention span
2. Behavior problems associated with hyperactivity
3. Combined hyperkinetic behavior and learning disorders with underachieving, reading and speech difficulties, impaired motor coordination, and impulsive/compulsive behavior, often described as asocial, antisocial, or delinquent

In 1983 Riker discontinued making Deaner because the FDA asked for an efficacy study. An efficacy study would give more solid proof of the effectiveness of the drug in producing the above-listed results. Since the market was too small to make the costs of such a study worthwhile, Riker decided to drop the product.

The learning and behavior problems mentioned above are usually childhood disorders (but may be seen in adults) and are frequently treated with amphetamine or amphetamine-like drugs. DMAE represents a safe alternative treatment for these problems. In a large study (eighty-three boys and twenty-five girls), 76 percent of the girls had fair to good improvement in their behavior and 66 percent of the boys had similar improvement.

Overall, the children on Deaner therapy showed a decrease in hyperactivity, a lengthened attention span, decreased irritability, better scholastic ability and, in some cases, an increase in I.Q.[2]

The administration of DMAE increases the concentration of choline in the blood.[3] DMAE is able to cross the blood-brain barrier, but whether or not it directly raises the level of acetylcholine in the brain has not been proved conclusively. Some studies have shown that DMAE raises acetylcholine levels in the brain and others have not found this effect. This may be due to differences in the dosage levels and experimental design.

Although DMAE produces a mild stimulant effect, it differs significantly from the stimulation produced by amphetamines and amphetamine-like drugs. The stimulation from DMAE develops slowly over a period of two weeks. Reports from volunteer subjects indicate that after taking DMAE regularly for three to four weeks, the mild stimulation is continually present, without side effects. Also, no drug-like letdown or depression occurs when deanol is discontinued.[4]

The learning and behavior problems in children and some of the neurological problems in elderly people are believed to be the result of low levels of acetylcholine.[5,6] This probably explains why deanol and other precursors to acetylcholine can provide beneficial results for some people.

One DMAE study stated that total oral doses as low as 10 to 20 mg per day will produce a mild and pleasant degree of central nervous system stimulation within seven to ten days. There was less daytime fatigue, sounder sleep at night, and a decrease in the amount of sleep needed each night.[7]

Clinical Trial

In one of the earliest documented studies, Dr. Carl Pfeiffer reported that the best results obtained with DMAE therapy were in the treatment of patients with chronic fatigue and mild to moderate depression. In one study with over a hundred patients, DMAE produced an increase in drive and physical energy as well as improvements in personality and greater ease of sleep for people with insomnia. Dependency or tolerance did not develop and most patients spontaneously discontinued the medication as they felt better.[8]

A clinical trial conducted with young, healthy human subjects produced valuable results.[9] DMAE was compared to an identical-appearing placebo tablet under double-blind test conditions.

The dose was regulated at one tablet per day for the first week and two tablets per day for the second week. After two weeks the subjects were allowed to increase or decrease their daily dosage with the top limit set at three tablets per day. Treatment was continued for a six-week period during which time seventeen subjects received deanol and eighteen subjects received placebo therapy. After six weeks the double-blind portion of the experiment was terminated. All subjects were then placed on DMAE therapy and the experiment was continued for an additional six-week period.

Analysis: The First Six Weeks. After the first six weeks, the subjects taking DMAE showed an overall improvement in muscle tone. The DMAE group also had an increase in their ability for mental concentration. DMAE produced changes in sleep habits. In most instances less sleep was required. Others reported sleeping sounder, waking earlier, and having a clearer mind upon awakening.

Analysis: The Second Six Weeks. During the second six weeks, twenty-five of the thirty-five subjects noted a definite stimulant effect. Most subjects who noted stimulation with deanol reported greater daytime energy, attentiveness at lectures (but greater intolerance of poor lecturers), sounder sleep with a reduction in the hours of sleep needed, and better ability to concentrate on the writing of papers or studying. The usual apprehension before and during examinations was noticeably decreased.

Many reported a more affable mood and outspoken personality. Two subjects reported that they were able to stop smoking without difficulty, whereas previous attempts had been unsuccessful. Several subjects noted an increase in their tolerance to alcoholic beverages and freedom from "hangover" depression or headache.

Life Extension

DMAE is one of the memory-enhancing drugs that seems to also have tremendous potential in the area of life extension.[10] The health of the brain and the health of the body are intimately connected, so it is not surprising to find that some of the drugs that enhance mental capabilities and prevent or reverse the aging of the brain have a similar effect on our general health. Programs for optimal health naturally lead to life extension.

DMAE attracted attention as a drug with potential in the field of life extension because of its structural similarity to Lucidril, a drug with known life-extension properties. (The beneficial effects of Lucidril are discussed in Chapter 11.)

Cellular membrane degradation (the destruction of cellular membranes) has been proposed as a prime mechanism of aging. DMAE is common to a number of drugs known to stabilize cellular membranes.[11]

DMAE also increases the levels of choline in the blood because it enhances the rate at which free choline enters the blood from other tissues. It easily penetrates the blood-brain barrier and serves to raise the choline level in the brain, which increases the synthesis of acetylcholine. The way DMAE functions with choline to raise blood plasma levels of free choline is not yet fully understood. It is possible that DMAE works with dietary choline or lecithin to enhance levels of acetylcholine in the brain.

Gerovital (GH-3)

DMAE and the drug Gerovital have some similarities in their chemical structures and in their effects. Gerovital (also called procaine) is another drug whose antiaging and intelligence-enhancing effects are well known throughout the world. The main ingredient in Gerovital is procaine. Procaine is broken down in the body into the B vitamin PABA (para-aminobenzoic acid) and diethylaminoethanol (DEAE).

procaine   PABA

  or   ➡   +

Gerovital   diethylaminoethanol (DEAE)

The DEAE half of the Gerovital molecule is very similar to the structure of DMAE (deanol). With such similar structures, it is not surprising that they have some similar biological effects.

DMAE/DEANOL   DEAE

CH_3 CH_3-CH_2
  \   \
  $N-CH_3-CH_2OH$ $N-CH_3-CH_2OH$
  /   /
CH_3 CH_3-CH_2

DMAE is known for its effects as a mental stimulant whereas Gerovital is known for its antiaging function. It is not known if DEAE, one of the components of Gerovital, has the same effects on choline levels and mental energy as DMAE.

Side Effects

A large initial dosage of DMAE can produce dull headaches. Continued overdosage can produce tenseness in the muscles of the neck, jaw, legs, and other muscles. Overdosage can produce insomnia. No serious side effects have ever been reported with DMAE therapy. Minor side effects, if encountered, usually disappear with continued treatment or with reduction in dosage.

Older people often show a response pattern to a drug or nutrient different from that of a younger person. This should be considered carefully before starting any type of drug or nutrient therapy program. Generally it is safer to start off at lower dosages and gradually build up to higher levels if desired and as tolerated.

Usually older people can tolerate larger doses of DMAE than younger people. There are three possible contributing factors: (1) older people generally have lower brain levels of acetylcholine, (2) they may have reduced receptor sensitivity to acetylcholine, or (3) they may have altered feedback in brain metabolism.

Toxicity

The toxicity of DMAE is very low. Laboratory tests and clinical studies have not disclosed any harmful changes attributable to the drug.

Contraindications

No absolute contraindications are known for DMAE. However, patients with certain types of epilepsy should be monitored closely by a physician.

How Supplied

DMAE is available in most health food stores in the following forms:

1. *DMAE bulk powder*—available as the bitartrate salt on a nonprescription basis (Vitamin Research Products, Appendix B).
2. *DMAE capsules*—available on a nonprescription 100 basis in 40 mg and 100 mg strengths (in bottles of 100 or 500 capsules).
3. *DMAE liquid*—available in a 50 ml bottle in which ten drops contain 100 mg of DMAE.

Dosage Range

The manufacturer's package insert for Deaner stated the following guidelines:

Starting dose: 500 mg daily. If satisfactory improvement occurs, the maintenance dosage will vary from 250 mg to 500 mg daily, which should be adjusted to the needs of the individual patient.

A survey of the professional literature shows a wide dosage range for Deaner and/or DMAE. Pfeiffer reported effective results in a clinical trial giving volunteer medical students dosages of 10 mg to 30 mg daily.[12] Studies in children with either hyperkinetic behavior or learning disabilities report administering dosages ranging from 40 mg to 400 mg daily. Trials in adults with varying types of problems range from about 300 mg per day to as high as 6000 mg per day.[13]

The following information is from an article written by Dr. Osvaldo Re' titled:

"2-Dimethylaminoethanol Deanol:
A Brief Review of Its Clinical Efficacy
and Postulated Mechanism of Action."

1. Dosage: An average of 500 mg daily in children and 1000 mg daily in adults seems to be necessary for achieving clear-cut therapeutic effects. In some cases however, lower and/or individualized doses have resulted in satisfactory responses. Maximum daily dosage has not yet been established.

2. Length of Therapy: The best clinical effects have been achieved after three months of treatment in children and there seems to be a minimum period of time for best effects. Certainly no conclusions should be drawn as to success/failure before three weeks of therapy.[14]

In taking DMAE as well as with other intelligence-enhancing and antiaging therapies, the following point should be understood. The worse the impairment, the longer it may take to produce a noticeable improvement. On the other hand, greater impairment sometimes produces the quickest and most dramatic results. This paradox is another reason why it is safer to start with lower dosages and build up gradually to desired levels (under the direction of your health professional).

DMAE + Vitamin B-5

Compounds that are taken to enhance the production of the neurotransmitter acetylcholine (DMAE, choline, or lecithin) may be more effective if taken with additional amounts of vitamin B-5 (calcium pantothenate), which helps in the synthesis of acetylcholine.

More DMAE Research Needed

The destruction of cellular membranes is known to be one of the primary mechanisms of aging. DMAE is part of the structure of many drugs that are known to stabilize membranes. Choline is a vital part of the cellular membrane and DMAE is the immediate precursor of choline in the building and repair of cellular membranes. Further research is needed to clarify the extent of DMAE's ability to prevent the aging of cellular membranes and its effect on acetylcholine supplies in the brain for optimal memory and learning.

9

Hydergine:
The Ultimate Smart Pill

Hydergine is probably the most important smart pill available in the United States today. It acts in several different ways to enhance mental capabilities and slow down or reverse the aging processes in the brain. The major effects of this important drug are listed below:

1. Increases blood supply to the brain.
2. Increases the amount of oxygen delivered to the brain.
3. Enhances metabolism in brain cells.
4. Protects the brain from damage during periods of decreased and/or insufficient oxygen supply.
5. Slows the deposit of age pigment (lipofuscin) in the brain.
6. Prevents free radical damage to brain cells.
7. Increases intelligence, memory, learning, and recall.

Hydergine is a mixture of three different ergot alkaloids. These alkaloids come from a fungus (*Claviceps purpurea*) that grows naturally on rye and other grains. In Europe, the Sandoz Pharmaceutical Company contracts for massive fields of rye to be grown. The fungus is separated from the grain at the time of harvest. So Hydergine is derived from a natural, organic source. However, after the alkaloid is removed and isolated, a couple of chemical steps are needed to change the alkaloids into the form used in the Hydergine formula. The specific alkaloids in Hydergine were chosen because of their high level of biological activity and the unique healing properties they have. Hydergine is called a semisynthetic because of the chemical steps necessary to change the alkaloids into their final form.

Hydergine and Senility

Hydergine was initially introduced as a treatment for senility (senile dementia). Many of the symptoms of senility are thought to be due to hardening of the arteries in the brain, which leads to poor blood supply and a shortage of oxygen in the brain. The FDA has approved the use of hydergine only as a treatment for senile dementia and related circulatory problems.

Some of the symptoms of senile dementia are: decreased mental alertness, confusion, problems with orientation, loss of memory of recent events, forgetfulness, depression, emotional instability, dizziness, and problems with walking and motor skills. Those suffering from senile dementia can develop any one or a combination of these symptoms.

The effectiveness of Hydergine for the treatment of senile dementia has been tested in a great many studies in the last ten to fifteen years. A comprehensive review of twenty-two well-controlled double-blind studies showed a significant improvement in the Hydergine-treated patients in all of the studies.[1]

Another important factor emerged from the review of this scientific research. In all cases, those patients who received higher doses of Hydergine (4.5 mg to 6 mg/day) showed the greatest improvement. It is important to understand the significance of this point. In the United States, the FDA has limited the approved dosage level of Hydergine to 3 mg/day, whereas in Europe the approved dosage level is three times higher (9 mg/day). All the research shows that the higher dosage levels are *more* effective in cases of senility.

The U.S. dosage of 3 mg/day was shown to be insufficient for many patients with cerebrovascular disease. More patients showed clinically significant improvement at the higher dosage levels. Another important point is that no serious side effects are produced at either dosage level. Therefore, the research reports that the higher dosages are more effective, without the risk of side effects.

Hydergine produces improvements that are statistically significant in patients suffering from senile dementia, but it does not produce miracles. A large number of patients show a relatively small amount of improvement, whereas only a few patients obtain major improvement.[2,3] Hydergine is of greater benefit in patients with mild to moderate mental deterioration, and therapy should be initiated as soon as possible. Delay only reduces the chance of a good response.

As mentioned previously, so far the only uses for Hydergine approved by the Food and Drug Administration are the treatment of senile dementia and cerebrovascular insufficiency (poor blood circulation to the brain). However, research in other countries has shown that Hydergine increases mental abilities, prevents damage to brain cells, and even may be able to reverse existing damage to the brain cells. This information is not readily available in the United States.

Hypoxia

Oxygen is unique in that it is both a free radical generator and a free radical scavenger. The term hypoxia means an inadequate supply of oxygen. When the oxygen supply to individual tissues and cells is optimal, the rate of free radical generation by oxygen is balanced by its ability to neutralize free radicals, and little if any damage results. An inadequate supply of oxygen to the brain upsets this balance, which allows the production of more free radicals.

The net effect of a decreased supply of oxygen to the brain is a significant increase in free radicals and free radical-generated damage to brain cells. Free radical-induced damage to the fatty acids in the brain is probably the major cause of progressive aging of the brain.

88   IMPROVING PERFORMANCE

A reduced supply of oxygen can cause damage to many parts of the body. Here are some examples:

1. Heart attacks usually result in some damage to the heart muscle because there has been a lack of blood supply to part of the heart. The decreased blood supply means less oxygen (hypoxia), which increases the level of free radicals and results in physical damage to the heart muscle.

2. A stroke is a rupture in a blood vessel in the brain. A large part of the damage from such an event (partial paralysis, loss of speech, etc.) is due to free radical damage.

3. Smoking cigarettes is a major cause of free radical damage. Smoking is not just a double whammy. It's a triple whammy. There are three different ways that smoking contributes to increased free radical damage.

    a. The carbon monoxide in smoke greatly reduces the oxygen-carrying capacity of the blood.

    b. The nicotine from smoking constricts the blood vessels, which decreases the supply of oxygen to the brain.

    c. The high temperatures at the burning tip of a cigarette produce substances that are carcinogenic and potent free radical generators.

What effect does cigarette smoking have on the brain? Dr. R. L. Rogers and his colleagues at the Baylor College of Medicine in Houston studied this problem. They published the results of their research in a paper titled: "Non-smokers Are Smarter."[4]

They found that individuals who smoke more than a pack a day lose at least 7 percent of the normal blood flow to the brain. This is exactly the type of oxygen imbalance that causes a tremendous increase in the number of free radicals and in the amount of free radical damage to the brain. Smokers as a group would probably receive substantial protection from Hydergine.

The Cat Experiment

An important experiment into the ability of Hydergine to prevent brain damage has been overlooked, possibly because it was conducted in Europe. In the experiment two groups of cats were anesthetized and their brain waves were electronically monitored. Researchers reduced the brain's blood supply (and oxygen) to a critical level. The control group (i.e.) non-Hydergine treated cats) began to show evidence of brain damage within five minutes. After fifteen minutes, the cats in the control group had suffered massive, irreversible brain damage and were essentially dead.

The same experiment was conducted with cats that were pretreated with Hydergine. The monitoring equipment showed no indication of any brain damage at the five-minute mark. After fifteen minutes, these cats still showed strong brain wave readings. After forty-five minutes, the Hydergine treated cats *still* had normal brain energies and no detectable brain damage![5]

The cat experiment dramatically demonstrates the following points:

1. A decrease in the normal oxygen balance results in tremendous free radical-generated damage to the brain.
2. Hydergine protects against and prevents free radical damage when the oxygen balance is upset.

These results underline Hydergine's potential for protecting people from the brain damage and paralysis that often occurs in stroke victims.

Saving Lives

Hydergine is used regularly in many European countries in emergencies such as accidents with shock or hemorrhage, strokes and heart attacks, drowning, electrocution, and drug overdose. There are reports of accident victims who were thought to be dead and were then revived by quick intravenous administration of Hydergine.

Hospitals in Europe routinely give Hydergine to many patients before standard operations. Medical staffs have more time to deal with any ensuing crisis during an operation if the patient has been pretreated with Hydergine.

How Hydergine Works

Early research in patients with senile dementia documented Hydergine's ability to increase the blood supply (and oxygen) to brain tissues. It was assumed that Hydergine was dilating the blood vessels of the brain. Recent research has shown that this is not the case, and that several other mechanisms are involved:

1. Hydergine is now thought to stimulate behavior by increasing the level of some neurotransmitters in the brain.[6]

2. Hydergine improves brain metabolism. This important effect is produced by keeping several neurotransmitters in proper balance. A deepening understanding of Hydergine's effect on cell metabolism has provided an explanation for the improvement Hydergine produces in oxygen utilization, blood flow, and brain wave activity.[7,8]

3. A substance called nerve growth factor (NGF) stimulates protein synthesis that results in the growth of dendrites in brain cells. Dendrites facilitate communication throughout the central nervous system and are necessary for memory and learning. New learning requires new dendritic growth. There is evidence that Hydergine may be able to stimulate the growth of dendrite nerve fibers in the same way as NGF although this mechanism is not yet well understood.[9]

Hydergine decreases the rate at which age pigment (lipofuscin) accumulates in the brain.[10] This is probably due to a combination of Hydergine's ability to enhance brain cell metabolism and its powerful antioxidant properties that greatly reduce the amount of free radical damage that occurs.

Hydergine is authorized for the treatment of senility and similar age-related disorders. However, some research has shown that better results are achieved in patients with mild to moderate mental deterioration as compared to severe cases. It is a powerful antioxidant that protects the brain against free radical damage, which slows down brain aging.

Research has established that higher dosages of Hydergine are more effective, are virtually nontoxic, and are without side effects, even at dosage levels that are higher than the FDA-approved level of 3 mg/day. The suggested dosage level in Europe is 9 mg/day, which is three times higher than in the U.S.A.[11]

Hydergine's Effects on Healthy People

We have established that many elderly people suffering from senile deterioration may benefit from taking Hydergine. Now we will examine Hydergine's effect on healthy people. The following two studies address this question.

1. A study in England monitored the performance of ten normal volunteers taking 12 mg of Hydergine per day over a two week period.[12] Note that the 12 mg/day dosage is four times greater than the approved U.S. dosage. This high dose of Hydergine was well tolerated by all subjects. A variety of tests were used to assess mental performance. The results indicated that Hydergine produced significant improvement in both simple alertness and high-level cognitive function in young, healthy volunteers.

2. Another important Hydergine study recently reported in the professional literature is titled: "A Controlled Long-term Study with Ergoloid Mesylates (Hydergine) in Healthy, Elderly Volunteers: Results After Three Years."

This long-term clinical trial is currently being conducted. The study compares the effects of Hydergine against a placebo on 148 healthy, elderly volunteers of both sexes and carries special significance. Most Hydergine studies have been short-term (about twelve weeks) investigations of aging, demented (unhealthy) subjects. This contemporary study breaks important new ground in that it is studying the benefits from the long-term administration of Hydergine to healthy people.[13]

The study has a fairly large number of subjects—148. A

significant trend with this many subjects could make a statistically meaningful statement. In fact, the results at the three-year point in this study do show a trend. The study demonstrated the following results:

1. The administration of Hydergine on a long-term basis is well tolerated. No side effects and no adverse changes were observed.

2. Systolic blood pressure was normalized (significantly lowered in those subjects with high initial values, but increased in subjects with low initial values).

3. Heart rate increased significantly in subjects with low initial values (by 5 beats/min on average).

4. Hydergine produced improvements in electrical brain wave measurements.

5. The number of subjects with abnormal cholesterol levels decreased significantly in the Hydergine group.

6. Subjective symptoms—i.e., tiredness, dizziness, tinnitus (ringing in the ears), visual disturbances, etc.—*decreased* in the Hydergine group during the three years of the trial but *increased* in the placebo group.

7. Hydergine may produce a favorable effect on the maintenance of cognitive functions (learning and memory).

None of these findings taken in isolation is evidence of a dramatic effect of Hydergine on the elderly volunteers. Taken together, however, the findings produce a pattern indicating that Hydergine, taken regularly over three years by physically and mentally healthy elderly people, helped them to maintain their physical and mental health and reflected this in terms of fewer subjective complaints and increased general well-being.

The collective results indicate that: *Hydergine slows down the aging process!*

Hydergine was definitely able to retard important signs and symptoms of aging in the subjects (the brain wave findings support this claim). The study is still in progress, and the expectation is that the favorable results observed after three years will be maintained.

Classification

Hydergine is a prescription drug. The FDA has authorized its use in the United States to treat elderly individuals who begin to show the signs and symptoms of senile dementia, which is the loss or impairment of mental powers associated with aging.

Hydergine comes from a family of drugs called the ergot alkaloids, which are well known for their wide range of pharmacological effects. Two generic terms for this product are ergoloid mesylates and dihydrogenated ergot alkaloids.

Side Effects

One of the exciting things about Hydergine therapy is that it does not produce any serious side effects. There have been occasional reports of sublingual irritation, slight nausea, gastric disturbance, and headache, but these are uncommon and usually the result of taking large doses to start, rather than gradually building up to the higher dosage levels.

Toxicity

Hydergine is virtually nontoxic. Even in studies experimenting with dosage levels four times higher than allowed in the United States, there was no toxicity observed in any of the subjects.[14]

Contraindications

Hydergine is contraindicated in patients who have chronic or acute psychosis, regardless of the origin because it could lead to a worsening of the condition.

How Hydergine Is Supplied

Hydergine was originally manufactured and marketed by Sandoz Pharmaceuticals. The marketing and distribution of Hydergine are now handled by Dorsey Pharmaceuticals. Although Dorsey is a division of Sandoz, the product still carries the Sandoz trademark. It is available in several different strengths and dosage forms.

1. *Hydergine sublingual tablets:*

   a. 0.5 mg strength are round white tablets, embossed with HYDERGINE 0.5 on one side and the Sandoz company logo on the other side; supplied in bottles of 100 and 1000.

   b. 1.0 mg strength are oval, white tablets, embossed with HYDERGINE on one side and 78-77 on the other side; supplied in bottles of 100 and 1000.

2. *Hydergine oral tablets:*

   1.0 mg oral tablets are round, white, and embossed with HYDERGINE 1 on one side and the Sandoz logo on the other side; supplied in bottles of 100 and 500.

3. *Hydergine liquid:*

   1.0 mg/ml strength, in bottles containing 100 ml with a dropper graduated to deliver a 1 mg dose.

4. *Hydergine liquid capsules:*

   1.0 mg oblong, off-white capsules, branded "Hydergine 1 mg" on one side and having the Sandoz company logo on the other side.

The liquid capsule is the newest dosage form in the Hydergine product line. It was approved and made available to the public in the fall of 1983.

When Hydergine is taken orally, much of it is destroyed in the stomach and/or the liver. The Sandoz company reports that the liquid capsules produce a 12 percent greater bioavailability (available to the body) than the oral tablets.

Generic Brands

Manufacturers secure exclusive rights to new products by applying for a patent. A patent gives exclusive rights to the patent holder to make, use, license, and market a product for seventeen years. After the patent expires, other manufacturers are free to begin producing and marketing the product under the generic name. The cost of generic drugs is usually significantly lower than the brand name product.

The Sandoz patent on Hydergine has expired. Consequently, generic brands of dihydrogenated ergot alkaloids are now available in some strengths.

Bolar Pharmaceutical Co., Inc., manufactures generic Ergoloid Mesylate tablets for direçt distribution and for sale to other generic drug companies. Both laboratory and clinical tests have been conducted on Bolar's Ergoloid Mesylate tablets. The FDA reviewed this material and issued an "AB" rating indicating the product is biologically equivalent to the original brand name product.[15]

Dosage Range

In the United States, the manufacturer's recommended daily dosage for Hydergine as approved by the FDA is 1 mg three times daily.

The manufacturer's product information and package insert state that "the alleviation of symptoms is usually gradual and results may not be observed for three to four weeks."

European Dosage

The following information is especially significant for Americans, who are restricted from having access to important advances in health and medical research from other countries. The recommended daily dosage for Hydergine in Europe is 3 mg taken three times daily.

Note that the recommended daily dosage in Europe is three times greater than in the United States. Many of the scientific research studies have been at levels closer to or higher than the European dosages. As previously mentioned, several studies have been published showing higher dosages of Hydergine produce significantly better results. Remember that it may be best to begin with a low dose and work up to higher doses to avoid possible mild side effects.

How to Obtain Hydergine

In the United States, Hydergine is only available as a prescription drug. Also, many doctor's may not be familiar with the intelligence enhancement and antiaging applications of this drug because FDA restrictions prevent drug companies from telling doctors about new (FDA unapproved) uses for their products.

Ask your doctor to write the prescription for 500 to 1000 tablets. If the prescription is written for a smaller quantity, ask the doctor to indicate PRN refills for six months or a year. PRN is a Latin abbreviation used on prescriptions that means "refill as needed."

Cost of Obtaining Hydergine

Listed below are the current average wholesale prices (AWP) for Hydergine as of October 1988.

Hydergine 0.5 mg sublingual tablets	$28.02/100
Hydergine 0.5 mg sublingual tablets	$265.02/1000
Hydergine 1.0 mg sublingual tablets	$53.28/100
Hydergine 1.0 mg sublingual tablets	$501.00/1000
Hydergine 1.0 mg oral tablets	$44.28/100
Hydergine 1.0 mg oral tablets	$209.04/500
Hydergine 1.0 mg Liquid Capsules	$35.76/100
Hydergine 1.0 mg Liquid Capsules	$168.00/500
Hydergine Liquid in 100 ml bottles	$36.54/bottle

I strongly suggest that you shop and compare prices when having prescriptions filled. The price of this drug can cost twice as much at some pharmacies. It is to your benefit to check prices before having your prescriptions filled.

Generic Prices

A pharmacy has to increase the price it charges for a drug over the acquisition price (wholesale) cost to make a profit. Usually the price is increased by a factor of two or more. The following prices represent average acquisition costs for pharmacies on generic Hydergine as of October, 1988.

Generic 0.5 mg sublingual tablets	$8.35/100
Generic 0.5 mg sublingual tablets	$25.20/500
Generic 1.0 mg sublingual tablets	$9.20/100
Generic 1.0 mg sublingual tablets	$17.96/250
Generic 1.0 mg oral tablets	$14.80/100
Generic 1.0 mg oral tablets	$106.35/1000

Mail Order

Hydergine and a number of other intelligence-enhancing drugs mentioned in this book may be available by mail from: Pharmaceuticals International. See Appendix B for an explanation of the situation regarding the ordering of intelligence drugs from mail order sources.

Final Comments

The following are some statistics that give added insight into how widely used and accepted Hydergine is on a worldwide basis.

1. For several years during the 1970s, Hydergine was the fifth most popular drug in the world. In 1982, Hydergine was ranked sixth.
2. For several years, Hydergine was the number one prescription drug in all of France.

3. Statistics in the pharmaceutical industry indicated that in one recent year Hydergine accounted for over $300,000,000 in sales.

Hydergine is one of the most widely studied drugs in the world, with over three thousand research papers published on its effects. However, there is a definite need for more research into its benefits in the areas of intelligence enhancement and antiaging effects. There has not been enough research on determining the optimal individual dosage levels, and more research is needed on the long-term benefits and effects. Such studies would establish whether the initial improvements are maintained over a period of time.

Hopefully through this research the positive effects of Hydergine will become more widely known in the United States so that it will be more easily available to those who want to use it.

10
Vasopressin/Diapid: The Memory Hormone

What is your most vivid memory? Everyone has pictures in their mind and clear memories of the major events in their lives, such as weddings, surprises, and traumatic incidents. The reason memories such as these are so vividly etched in your mind is that your brain was bathed in vasopressin at the time.

Vasopressin is actually a brain hormone that is released by the pituitary gland and helps incorporate new information into your memory. Vasopressin facilitates more effective learning by helping to "imprint" new information in the memory centers of the brain. Learning, or the acquisition of new information, cannot be achieved without the action of vasopressin.

Vasopressin also helps retrieve information from your memory. It seems that when you try to recall information, vasopressin helps you "search" your memory and then withdraw or retrieve the desired information back into your consciousness.

Vasopressin is available as a prescription drug called Diapid. In recent years vasopressin has become widely known for its ability to enhance memory and recall. As a result, Diapid has become an important addition to the growing class of memory-improving drugs. The vasopressin in Diapid is synthetically produced, but it is exactly the same as the memory-stimulating hormone in your brain.

Effects

One of vasopressin's functions is the regulation of urine volume and serum electrolytes. Doctors usually prescribe Diapid nasal spray for those who do not produce enough natural vasopressin. This is the only application for Diapid that has been authorized by the FDA.

Clinical studies in both Europe and the United States have shown that:

1. Vasopressin produces a substantial improvement in both short-term and long-term memory.
2. Vasopressin improves performance on tests involving attention, concentration, retention, recognition, and recall.
3. Vasopressin enhances memory and learning abilities in some memory-impaired patients and in normally aging individuals.
4. Vasopressin has produced positive results in some patients with long histories of severe depression.

Vasopressin and Memory

The role of vasopressin in memory and learning was discovered by Dr. David de Wied at the University of Utrecht in the Netherlands. As early as 1965, he began to research, discover, and publish reports showing the effects of vasopressin on learning and memory in experimental animals. By 1969, de Wied reported that vasopressin improved long-term memory and had a role in the memory retrieval process.

He postulated that vasopressin induces changes within the brain and central nervous system that help transform the electrical impulses of learning into chemically encoded long-term memories. The final step of the process, in which memories are "imprinted," appears to involve the actual synthesis of new proteins that are then deposited in cells in selected areas of the brain.[1]

Other studies by de Wied have shown that vasopressin administered to laboratory animals will:

1. Facilitate memory retention.
2. Ease the acquisition of active learned behavior.
3. Protect against memory loss due to chemical or physical injury.
4. Reverse amnesia.
5. Reverse the severe memory disturbance in animals with congenital deficiencies of vasopressin hormone.[2]

Many researchers have investigated the new applications of vasopressin in the area of memory and learning. Several clinical trials and experiments have led to a new understanding of vasopressin's potential. In one case a fifty-five-year-old man with serious head injuries from an automobile accident was suffering from amnesia. After five days of treatment with vasopressin, he showed remarkable progress. His general mood improved dramatically and he regained his memory.

In another case a twenty-one-year-old could not remember anything that had happened to him in the three months before and after a severe car accident. After only one day of vasopressin treatment, he could recall some details of the accident. By the seventh day he had recovered his memory completely. His mood improved and he began to sleep well for the first time since the accident.[3]

A study of patients aged fifty to sixty tested the effects of vasopressin on learning ability, memory, and speed of muscle response. One group was given vasopressin three times a day for three days. The other group received a placebo. The patients who received vasopressin did better on tests of attention, concentration, and speed of muscle response. They also did better than the control group on the memory tests.[4]

The National Institutes of Mental Health (NIMH) found that depressed patients had lower levels of vasopressin in the cerebrospinal fluid. They gave vasopressin to four severely depressed patients and closely monitored their behavior and memory. This research studied both short- and long-term memory. The study showed that vasopressin significantly improved the overall short-term memory in three of the four patients, and the performance of long-term memory nearly doubled.[5]

One patient in the study had experienced delusions and hallucinations almost continuously for six months before treatment. Within forty-eight hours after the vasopressin therapy began, the depression began to lift, and after three weeks she showed continuing reduction in the depression. Also, the hallucinations had almost completely stopped.

Use of Vasopressin in Humans

Following the early work of de Wied with laboratory animals, many human studies and case reports with vasopressin have been published. These initial human studies were done with patients who were suffering from posttraumatic amnesia, amnesia due to alcoholism, and other types of memory disorders. Results from these initial human trials were often astounding.

Some of the first tests involved patients with long standing amnesia due to serious head injuries from automobile accidents. The administration of vasopressin produced remarkable recoveries within several days. Several people started showing signs of recovery within hours after the first dose.[6]

Studies on Healthy Subjects

Dr. Legros, at the University of Liège in Belgium, reported that vasopressin may be able to improve attention and memory in humans and restore lost memory associated with normal aging. Patients receiving vasopressin performed better on tests involving attention, concentration, motor rapidity, visual retention, recognition, recall, and learning.[7]

One study of young, healthy subjects (college volunteers) documented the effects of vasopressin on memory. One group of students was given vasopressin and the other was given a placebo. The subjects treated with vasopressin demonstrated significant increases in learning ability and memory.

A study in Hungary showed that treatment of healthy individuals with vasopressin led to an improvement in both short- and long-term memory.[8] The researchers indicate that vasopressin may improve memory function by a direct action on the central nervous system.

In the United States at the National Institutes for Mental Health (NIMH), scientists tested the effects of a vasopressin analog on healthy college students. In every case, the subjects were able to recall longer sequences of words when receiving vasopressin.[9]

Vasopressin and Recreational Drugs

Stimulant recreational drugs, such as cocaine, LSD, amphetamines, and the prescription drugs Ritalin and Cylert, cause a release of vasopressin. Frequent use of stimulant drugs will deplete the brain's supply of vasopressin. This leads to depression and a noticeable decrease in mental ability. These effects are most dramatic when seen in a typical cocaine user, who is very slow and sluggish in mental performance. Heavy cocaine users cannot express themselves well and often are so "spaced out" they appear to be walking around in a fog.

While stimulant drugs release vasopressin to the point of depletion, depressant drugs such as alcohol and marijuana inhibit the release of vasopressin. This may explain why regular users of these drugs have memory problems.[10]

Diapid produces a rapid transformation in many of these people because it is a direct application of the specific brain chemical that has been depleted. The effect and the improvement are almost immediate. As Diapid is inhaled, it is absorbed through the mucous membranes in the nasal passages and moved quickly to the brain.

The results are so fast and so impressive that both the Diapid user and first time observers are shocked at the spectacular transformation. You can see the change happening in less than a minute. It is as though a dense fog is lifting. Dull eyes start to sparkle; a smile often appears. Within minutes, the individual's mood, attitude, and expression improves.

Vasopressin/Best Uses

At this time there is no published research on long-term use of vasopressin. However, there is strong evidence indicating that Diapid is both safe and effective for short-term therapy in the following applications:

1. Older patients who begin to manifest the signs and symptoms of a decline in mental capacity
2. Fast, effective enhancement of short-term memory
3. Temporary amnesia from concussion, shock, or trauma

Amnesia due to alcoholism has also been treated successfully.

Other applications for vasopressin include situations where there is a large amount of new information to learn. For example, learning a new language is an excellent application for vasopressin. It increases your ability to memorize and recall the new vocabulary. Vasopressin also seems to help when studying for tests, especially when there is specific factual information that must be recalled.

Classification

Vasopressin is an actual brain hormone. It is used in three different forms: lysine-vasopressin or LVP, arginine-vasopressin (AVP), and 1-desamino-8-D-arginine or DDAVP. These different forms are just vasopressin with another molecule added on. For example, Diapid Nasal Spray (LVP) is vasopressin with the amino acid lysine chemically bound to it.

Research indicates that these different forms or analogs have similar if not identical activity and effects. Drug companies put forth two reasons for making these different analogs. They claim fewer side effects and a slight increase in potency.

I have not found any documentation to substantiate either of these claims. A third explanation may make more sense. The drug companies are making synthetic analogs of vasopressin so that they can have a specific product to patent and market.

Side Effects

Adverse reactions observed with Diapid in clinical use are infrequent and mild. These reactions include runny nose, nasal congestion, slight itch or irritation of the nasal passages, nasal ulceration, headache, abdominal cramps, and increased bowel movements. Generally speaking, research has shown Diapid to be very safe. No major side effects have been encountered.

Contraindications

There are no known contraindications to the use of Diapid Nasal Spray. The safety of Diapid in pregnancy has not been established.

How Supplied

Diapid Nasal Spray is manufactured by the Sandoz Pharmaceutical Company. It is supplied in a plastic bottle that contains 8 ml of solution. There are approximately 200 doses in one 8 ml bottle.

Dosage Range

One whiff of Diapid provides approximately 2.0 U.S.P. Posterior Pituitary Units. Most published human studies have used 12 to 16 units daily. This is equivalent to one spray to each nostril 3 to 4 times daily.

How to Obtain Diapid

Diapid is a prescription drug in the United States. Therefore, obtaining Diapid involves finding a doctor who is willing to write you a prescription for it. Many doctors may not be familiar with Diapid. The PDR only supplies a doctor with information regarding Diapid's use for diabetes insipidus. As mentioned earlier, diabetes insipidus is not a common medical problem. In fact, it is quite uncommon. Your doctor may never have had a patient with diabetes insipidus and he may not be familiar with Diapid Nasal Spray.

Diapid can also be ordered by mail order from Pharmaceuticals International (see Appendix B).

Cost of Obtaining Diapid

As of October 1988 the average wholesale price (AWP) for Diapid Nasal Spray was $27.00 per vial. The pharmacy will add the cost of having your prescription filled.

Final Comments

As with many drugs that may have intelligence-enhancing effects, there is a need for more research on the effects of vasopressin on healthy people. Research is now needed to determine ideal dosage levels and whether long-term usage leads to side effects or the development of tolerance. Furthermore, does vasopressin's memory-enhancing capability have any effect on preventing the loss of memory with aging?

There have been only a few studies on the ability of vasopressin to stimulate the acquisition of new learning. There is a definite need for more studies to enlarge our understanding of how vasopressin and other intelligence enhancing drugs produce their effects. We must begin to focus on the biochemistry of health instead of concentrating on drugs that cure diseases.

11

Lucidril: Reversing the Aging Process

Lucidril is one of the most promising new drugs in the areas of brain research and antiaging. It is widely used throughout Europe to prevent biological aging and reverse the aging process. Studies have shown that it removes age pigment deposits from brain cells. This is actually reversing part of the aging process. Human clinical trials with Lucidril have demonstrated improvements in memory and mental functioning.

The generic name for Lucidril is centrophenoxine. Throughout this book we will refer generally to this drug as Lucidril. It is interesting to note that the brand name for this drug is derived from the word "lucid," meaning clear-thinking.

Effects

Lucidril slows down the rate of accumulation of age pigment deposits (lipofuscin) in brain cells, and it also removes deposits that have already accumulated in aged brains.

1. Lucidril seems to improve the functioning of the central nervous system. It is not yet clear if this is a primary or secondary effect.

2. In clinical trials Lucidril has produced marked improvement in geriatric patients suffering from:

    a. Generalized weakness and loss of vigor
    b. Confusion
    c. Disturbances of memory and intellectual function
  3. Human clinical trials have shown that centrophenoxine improves long-term memory and increases mental alertness.

Cellular Garbage

There is an important relationship between the quantity of cellular garbage deposits and the rate of biological aging. Imagine how your personal life would change if you stopped throwing out your trash, garbage, and waste. Most of us would soon be submerged in a house full of unspeakable filth. The process would take longer if you only threw out part of your waste, but the end result would be much the same. Eventually you would be buried in your own waste.

We have a remarkably similar process to contend with at the cellular level. Normal cellular activities are constantly producing metabolic waste products. Without complete removal, metabolic wastes gradually accumulate inside individual cells. These waste deposits are called age pigment or lipofuscin. When lipofuscin deposits become visible on the surface of the skin, they are called age spots or liver spots.

Lipofuscin/Age Pigment

Neurons in certain areas of the brain are primary sites of lipofuscin accumulation. Initially the buildup of lipofuscin in brain cells shows little or no detrimental effect. However, with continual accumulation, lipofuscin increasingly clogs up the cell, inhibiting the flow of nutrients and enzyme activity. Several studies have reported a "threshold effect." When a certain level is reached, rapid deterioration of cellular function occurs, resulting in the eventual death of the cell.[1,2]

The fact that lipofuscin deposits accumulate in brain cells is frequently reported in scientific literature, but knowledge of its mode of origin is incomplete. Information from different investigators suggests several sources as probable contributors to the buildup of lipofuscin.

Some research suggests that mitochondria are associated with lipofuscin deposits. Mitochondria are the "power plants" within cells where oxygen and nutrients are transformed into energy. Incomplete removal of waste products from this metabolic activity may create lipofuscin.

Lysosomes are the waste disposal units in cells. They contain strong digestive enzymes to digest cellular waste and debris. Lipofuscin may accumulate if lysosomes become overloaded with cellular waste or if the lysosomal membranes become damaged, allowing the caustic enzymes to leak out into other areas of the cell.[3]

Demopoulos and other investigators suggest that lipofuscin deposits may be accumulated debris from free radical attacks that damage cell membranes and cellular components.[4]

The most striking characteristic of Lucidril is its ability to reduce deposits of lipofuscin in laboratory animals. There is good reason to believe this extends to humans, but it must be emphasized that this is speculative (it is hard to find human volunteers who are willing to sacrifice their brains for a research study).

As early as 1966, Kalidas Nandy reported that treatment with Lucidril produced a notable decrease of lipofuscin deposits in most parts of the central nervous system. The degree of the reduction was largely dependent upon the duration of the treatment; the longer the administration of Lucidril, the greater the reduction of lipofuscin deposits.[5]

The electron microscope has made it possible for scientists to observe the actual clearing inside a cell as the lipofuscin is removed with centrophenoxine treatment.

Other studies have confirmed the age-related pigmentation deposits in nerve cells and Lucidril's ability to reduce these levels. The Biochemistry Institute in Bucharest, Romania, reported reductions of lipofuscin ranging from 25 percent to 42.3 percent in the treated animals. This represented a reversal to levels as low as those found only in very young animals.[6]

Improved Learning and Memory

After Kalidas Nandy discovered that Lucidril could remove lipofuscin from nerve cells in mice, he sought to determine if this in turn would produce any improvement in mental performance. He designed a study to test the effects of Lucidril on learning and memory in old mice, and correlated the results with changes in the lipofuscin age pigment in the brain of the treated animals.

The results showed that the Lucidril-treated, older mice scored almost as well as the young, untreated controls. The treated animals also showed significant reductions in lipofuscin levels in the brain.[7]

Rejuvenating Brain Cells

At the Verzar International Laboratory for Experimental Gerontology in Italy, Dr. Giuli and his associates observed that the connections between brain cells in the rat brain deteriorate markedly between eighteen and twenty-eight months of age (about forty-five to seventy years in human terms). This connection is called a synapse. The synapse is where nerve impulses pass from the axon (transmitter) of one cell to the dendrites (receivers) of another cell.

The Italian scientists knew about synaptic deterioration with age, and they were also aware that Lucidril has a general stimulating effect on the metabolism of nerve cells. With this in mind, they designed a study to look at the effects of Lucidril on synaptic deterioration. This study was published in 1980 in *Mechanisms of Aging and Development*. The results of this study are extremely exciting. They found that treatment with Lucidril restored the synaptic contact zones in brain cells of old rats to the values found in young animals.[8]

The rejuvenation of brain cells may be due to the strengthening of cellular membranes. This may result from an increased production of choline or from Lucidril's general stimulatory effect on the metabolism of nerve cells in the brain and central nervous system.

Memory Performance

The effects of Lucidril on memory performance were studied in a double-blind study with seventy-six elderly subjects who were all in good physical health, but suffered from a measurable amount of intellectual deterioration. The tests revealed that centrophenoxine appears to increase the storage of new information into long-term memory. Many of the subjects also reported an increased level of mental alertness.[9]

Classification

Chemically, centrophenoxine has two components. One half is a synthetic substance chemically related to the family of plant growth hormones called auxins. The second half is DMAE (Deanol), a naturally occurring precursor to the neurotransmitter acetylcholine (see Chapter 8). Several minutes after dissolving in water or in the stomach, centrophenoxine breaks down into its two components.

There has been no research that compares the effects of Lucidril and DMAE. Therefore, at this time, it has not been determined whether these two drugs duplicate each other's effects or if there are increased benefits from taking both.

Side Effects

The manufacturer's product information lists the following possible side effects for Lucidril:
1. Insomnia
2. Hyperexcitability

3. Tremor
4. Headache and/or dizziness
5. Sleepiness or depression

Adverse reactions with Lucidril have been infrequent and mild, but it is necessary to list the contraindications and possible side effects so that you are aware of them.

Contraindications

The manufacturer's product information lists the following contraindications for Lucidril:

1. Severe high blood pressure
2. Convulsive disorders
3. The lactation period for nursing mothers

Toxicity

There is virtually no toxicity with centrophenoxine in therapeutic doses.

How Supplied

Centrophenoxine is manufactured in tablet form for oral administration, and as an injectable. It is known by the following generic names: meclofenoxate, ANP 235, and clofenoxine. Commercially, it is sold under the trade names Lucidril and Helfergin. Lucidril is a 500 mg round, yellow tablet. It is packaged and sold with 20 foil-wrapped tablets to a box.

Dosage Range

The usual dosage of Lucidril administered in both animal and human clinical trials has been 80 mg/kg of body weight. For those people who are not familiar with the metric system, here are several examples that have been converted from the 80 mg/kg dosage to English equivalents:

WEIGHT	DAILY DOSAGE	TABLETS DAILY
120-pound person =	4.4 gm Lucidril =	9 tabs. daily
170-pound person =	6.2 gm Lucidril =	12 tabs. daily
220-pound person =	8.0 gm Lucidril =	16 tabs. daily
	(1 tablet = 500 mg)	

NOTE: These examples are included to provide a frame of reference between the dosages used in published studies and clinical trials, and English equivalents. In this book I am not recommending that you take any particular drug or dosage level. Let your physician be your guide to correct individual dosages.

Availability

Lucidril/centrophenoxine has not received approval from the FDA and consequently, it is not available in the United States.

Centrophenoxine is available from the following mail order source: Pharmaceuticals International (see Appendix B).

In Europe, centrophenoxine is also known as meclofenoxate, clofenoxine, and ANP 235, and is manufactured and marketed under the trade names Lucidril and Helfergin as 500 mg foil-wrapped tablets.

Summary

Life Extension. Lucidril has been shown to be effective as an intelligence drug and also in antiaging therapy. Research has clearly shown its ability to improve various aspects of memory function in both animals and humans. The fact that it has also produced a 30 percent increase in the life span of laboratory animals adds a fascinating dimension to this drug.[10]

Reversing Brain Aging. The accumulation of lipofuscin in brain cells is one of the most widely recognized aspects of aging. Lucidril removes lipofuscin deposits from aged brains and significantly reduces its rate of buildup in young, healthy animals. In doing so, it actually "rejuvenates" the synaptic structure—the area where the actual transfer of information takes place between nerve cells.[11] Much of the excitement about Lucidril is related to its apparent ability to actually reverse some aspects of the aging process and increase mental performance.

The way in which Lucidril removes lipofuscin deposits still is not understood fully. More research needs to be done to increase our knowledge of how it works, how early in life it would be beneficial to start taking Lucidril, and the length of treatment that produces maximum benefits. Also, it is hoped that Lucidril-like drugs will be available in the United States soon.

12

Dilantin/DPH: "A Remarkable Medicine Has Been Overlooked"

Diphenylhydantoin (DPH), also known as Dilantin, is a prescription drug commonly prescribed for epilepsy. It has also been found to be a versatile, remarkable medicine for the normalization and enhancement of mental functions. Research shows us that DPH improves concentration, learning, cognitive processes, and raises I.Q. DPH also has a stabilizing effect on disorders of the nervous system, cardiovascular system, and many other conditions.

When DPH was discovered in 1938, it was found to be the most effective anticonvulsant ever found. Its method of action is to stabilize or normalize unbalanced electrical activity in the brain. In fact, DPH stabilizes all cells that possess electrical activity.

Although DPH normalizes electrical activity that is out of balance, therapeutic doses do not adversely affect normal function. Thus, it can calm without sedation and improve energy without artificial stimulation. DPH is not habit-forming, and its levels of safety have been well established over the past forty years.

Exploration of Possible New Uses

It is exciting to become aware of the many types of disorders that can be helped with DPH. More than 2,200 studies on DPH are published in medical literature. These studies show that DPH is effective in the treatment of alcoholism, drug addiction, psychosis, pain, Parkinson's disease, asthma, diabetes, ulcers, hypertension, hypoglycemia, violent behavior, angina, as well as conditions related to thought, mood, and behavior. How can one substance be a remedy or treatment for such a wide range of disorders?

As previously mentioned, DPH stabilizes the electrical activity in our bodies, even at the level of the single cell. The most appropriate way to describe the function of DPH is to classify it as a "normalizer." It doesn't matter what area of the body is afflicted, when any area is out of balance electrically, DPH can help to normalize the malfunction.

At the cellular level, the human body is really an electrical machine. When we consider that all of our bodily functions are electrically regulated, our messages of pain are electrically transmitted, our memory processes are electrically stored and our thinking processes are electrically conducted, it makes it easier to understand DPH's breadth of use. Our understanding of the electrical nature of the body is also beginning to open up new avenues of therapy, treatment, and research.

Dr. Robert Becker, in his book *The Body Electric*, predicts a whole new era of science and medicine that centers around the relationship between electric currents and living things. It is well documented that electrical currents can speed up the healing of fractures and stimulate the immune system.

Biomagnetic therapy is beginning to be used in the treatment of cancer and other degenerative diseases. It seems that electromagnetic fields polarize the electrically charged components within cells, creating a greater level of intercellular organization, which improves function. Although this is not well understood yet, the effects have been demonstrated and well documented.

DPH and the Nervous System

DPH has beneficial effects on disorders of the nervous system, which often produce unfavorable personality characteristics. Most people have experienced or been exposed to irrational fits of anger, moodiness, depression, and irritability. When these conditions occur, the nervous system is most likely out of balance electrically.

DPH has even proved effective in treating some of the most violent personality disorders. In a study involving inmates in a prison, DPH caused significant improvement in conditions such as anger, fear, tension, impatience, impulsiveness, irritability, and hostility. In addition, improvements were observed in the prisoners related to other conditions such as sleep disorders, headaches, and gastrointestinal disturbances. In one case, phantom limb pain subsided.[1]

Subsequent observations were made on the effects of DPH on teenage juvenile delinquents at a reformatory. With a dose of only 100 mg daily, prompt relief in anger and fear were noted. This was clearly expressed in the marked decrease in fighting between the delinquents studied. Improvements in impatience, impulsiveness, tension, irritability, anger, fear sleep disorders and headaches were universally observed in the juveniles studied.[2]

A report was published in 1966 titled, "The Beneficial Effects of Diphenylhydantoin on the Nervous System of Nonepileptics—As Experienced and Observed in Others by a Layman." The author, Jack Dreyfus, observed that multiple simultaneous thoughts as well as obsessive and preoccupied thinking were relieved by DPH. Coincident with this relief, marked improvements were noted in symptoms of anger and the related conditions of impatience, irritability, agitation, and impulsiveness. Also coincident with the relief was marked improvement in fear and the related conditions of worry, pessimism, anxiety, apprehensiveness, and depression.[3]

DPH and Improved Cognitive Functions

DPH's ability to affect mental functions such as learning, concentration, and long-term memory is one of the most exciting areas for potential application. DPH is unique because it effectively improves cognitive processes without producing undesirable side or after effects. It stabilizes the nervous system without acting as either a stimulant or as a depressant.

Studies are showing that DPH assists in one's ability to concentrate by normalizing the overstimulated mind. How many times have you sat down to read or study, only to find your mind so cluttered with thoughts that it was impossible to concentrate? It is very difficult to bring in or process new information when undisciplined thoughts are dominating your mind.

In a study by Haward, published in the *International Journal of Neuropsychiatry*, the author concluded that "DPH improved concentration difficulties that seemed to stem from ruminative preoccupation with an irrelevant or nonessential thought content."[4]

A group of college students who had concentration difficulties were tested with DPH. Their performance in a complex task that produced fatigue was evaluated. The fatigue-producing task used for this study was a two-hour stint in an air traffic control simulator.

DPH was found to be significantly effective in delaying the onset of fatigue and accompanying errors. The author noted that although many substances have been used to improve concentration, these substances are usually stimulants. Use of DPH improved concentration significantly and produced none of the side effects of a stimulant.

These findings are in agreement with the observations of Dreyfus who speculated that poor concentration can result from forced ruminative thinking, or the "turned-on mind," and that this can be corrected by DPH.[5]

DPH and Improved I.Q.

In one study using normal healthy adults with no evidence of central nervous system disorders, standard I.Q. tests were used as a measurement standard. The test was administered on a double-blind crossover basis with placebo controls, and two retests were made. The authors reported "highly significant" increase in Verbal Scale and Full Scale intelligence scores, and "significant" increases on the Performance Scale.[6]

Another test assessed the mental functions of normal, healthy elderly persons. They were without specific complaints regarding mental functioning with intelligence levels ranging between normal and bright-normal. They represented middle and lower-upper socioeconomic classes. Intelligence tests were given before the trial with DPH and twice thereafter under double-blind drug and placebo conditions. The subjects showed significant increases in long-term memory and comprehension functions. They also showed an increase in the ability to learn new material and they also increased their speed of visual-motor coordination.[7]

Improving Mental Performance in the Elderly

In addition to the aforementioned study showing DPH's efficacy for elderly persons, there have been some animal experiments researching performance in the aged. In one such study, DPH was shown to improve deteriorated mental performance of older rats, but it did not affect normal behavior in young rats.[8] In another study, DPH facilitated learning on discrimination and avoidance tasks. The enhancement of performance in this study was more prominent among older rats. The authors of this study state that it is certainly possible that these findings have possible application to aging in humans.[9]

Jack Dreyfus

A discussion of DPH would not be complete without mentioning a man named Jack Dreyfus and the Dreyfus Medical Foundation. Mr. Dreyfus is a layman who had the good fortune to stumble on to Dilantin. He perceived a certain logic in trying Dilantin for his own problems, even though at the time, it was not known to be effective for his condition. He experienced incredible relief for what he considered a miserable condition. Over a period of several years he saw a number of other people get significant help from symptoms that were not listed as part of Dilantin's range or scope of effectiveness. It became apparent that Dilantin was effective for a wide variety of disorders that were virtually unknown to doctors.

Mr. Dreyfus decided he had a personal responsibility to bring Dilantin's new uses to the attention of the medical profession. In his private life Mr. Dreyfus had become a very successful businessman. This allowed him to create the Dreyfus Medical Foundation. He expected to spend $150,000 to $200,000 a year for two to three years to accomplish his task. The foundation ended up spending over $15 million over a period of fifteen years, without successfully completing the task.

Eventually Dreyfus published the book titled *A Remarkable Medicine Has Been Overlooked*. In the first section of his book Dreyfus tells background of his experiences and involvement with DPH. Part two contains clinical and scientific information. Two reports that had been published by the Dreyfus Medical Foundation titled *The Broad Range of Use of Diphenylhydantoin* (1970) and *DPH* (1975) are contained in this section, along with a review of recent work. This also includes a very complete bibliography that cites 2140 research studies on DPH.

Mr. Dreyfus opens the book with a letter to the President. In this open letter he tells the President that: "properties of a remarkable and versatile medicine are being overlooked," because of a flaw in the FDA's system of bringing medicines to the public.

The flaw, as he states it, is that it often takes as long as ten years and up to $50 million to bring a new drug to market. A company retains exclusive patent rights to a drug for seventeen years. When a patent expires, competition from other companies drives the price down and the incentive to do research on the drug is gone. If new uses for a drug are found, they are seldom developed because of time, money, and patent expiration conditions.

In my opinion, Mr. Dreyfus's assessment of the situation is accurate. That is why, besides Dilantin, such drugs as Hydergine and Diapid also fail to get recognized for other beneficial uses.

Side Effects and Toxicity

My approach in this book has been to only present substances that are virtually without side effects and toxicity. There are some significant side effects associated with DPH, but their occurrences seem to be fairly infrequent within the regular dosage range. Nausea, vomiting, headache, dizziness, tremor, and insomnia are side effects that can occur with DPH use. DPH can cause liver toxicity, but this effect occurs only rarely and if it occurs at all it is usually within the first few weeks.

DPH has also been reported to cause tenderness and excessive growth of gum tissue. This condition seems to have occurred most frequently in children with epilepsy who have been taking DPH regularly for a long time.

DPH can disturb the absorption of two essential vitamins, vitamin D and folic acid. Vitamin D is involved in the control of calcium in the body. Daily supplements of vitamin D, calcium, and folic acid will prevent and/or correct these problems.

Contraindications

The only contraindication for DPH is in the individual who has shown a previous hypersensitivity to this drug or other medications classified as hydantoins.

How Supplied

Dilantin is marketed and available in 100 mg capsules and 50 mg children's chewable tablets. Dilantin also comes in a liquid that contains 125 mg of Dilantin per teaspoonful.

Now that the original patent for Dilantin has expired, generic forms of the drug are available. Dilantin is known by two generic names, phenytoin and diphenylhydantoin (DPH). Although Dilantin is the trade name marketed in the United States, it is marketed in other countries as Epanutin, Epamin, Eplin, Idantoin, and Aleviatan.

Dosage Range

The adult dosage range for DPH is generally 100 mg, given two, three, or four times daily.

13

Cognitive Enhancers

The study of drugs that enhance memory, alertness, learning ability, and other aspects of human mental functioning is currently the most exciting area of pharmaceutical research. In fact, next to new cancer therapies, the quest for memory-improving drugs is the hottest area of medical research.

A completely new class of drugs, called the nootropics, is showing great promise in this area. The term nootropic comes from a Greek word meaning "acting on the mind." A number of similar terms are being coined to describe the activity of these drugs. They are being called cognitive enhancers, cognitive activators, performance enhancers, or just plain memory pills.

Nootropic drugs have unique effects on the central nervous system (CNS). They are not active in the classical pharmacological tests used to evaluate psychotropic drugs. They do not produce stimulation, sedation or analgesia, nor do they produce changes in the cardiovascular system or in overall behavior. They seem to be primarily active on tests in which learning and memory processes are involved. They are valuable also in treating impaired central nervous function as in cases of amnesia, anoxia, etc.

Structurally, the nootropics are derivatives of the neurotransmitter GABA, or gamma-aminobutyric acid. However, the nootropics do not seem to interact with the GABA pathways in the central nervous system, and as yet their mechanisms of action are not understood completely.

Nootropic drugs have the following properties in common:

1. They improve cognitive performances, especially on learning and memory tests.
2. They are especially effective at improving cognitive performance that is seen under conditions of disturbed nerve cell metabolism (such as hypoxia, trauma, intoxication, aging, etc.).
3. They have very minimal or essentially no side effects, even at very high doses.
4. They are able to cross the blood-brain barrier.
5. They have no vasoconstrictive or vasodilative activity.[1]

Piracetam, which will be discussed in depth in Chapter 14, was the first member of this new class of memory-enhancing drugs. It is now being marketed in over eighty-five countries throughout the world. Piracetam's worldwide success has set off many of the world's largest pharmaceutical companies on a virtual race to develop their own versions of these memory-enhancing drugs.

The pharmaceutical industry is not the only industry showing an interest in the development of these new drugs. The investment and banking communities are also keeping close tabs on what is happening. When these drugs successfully complete the maze of FDA testing regulations and become available in the United States, the financial gains could be enormous. Several companies are hoping to have their entry in the nootropic drug race on the market approved by the FDA by 1989. Financial analysts see the potential for a $1-billion-plus annual market for these drugs within just a few years.[2] The development and eventual sales of these cognitive enhancing drugs could surpass the successes of antibiotics and tranquilizers.

The nootropic drugs are presenting some interesting puzzles and challenges. Scientists do know they are effective in a variety of memory disorders, and that they enhance normal brain function in both animal and human experiments. The puzzle is that the researchers are not yet sure why these new drugs work or how they exert their effects. However, there is a good side to this "scientific frustration." It is forcing pioneering research in the biochemistry and physiology of intelligence and memory.

The search for the mechanism of action that produces the effects of nootropics is progressing on two fronts. First, the memory process itself has to be examined. Is the drug influencing the acquisition, consolidation, retention, retrieval, and/or interhemispheric transfer of memory? Second, we need to learn which physiological and biochemical processes are affected. Which neurotransmitters and/or receptor cites are involved? Are they being activated or inhibited? Which biochemical pathways are involved?

Thousands of scientific studies have been designed and published on memory-enhancing drugs in the past several years. This body of research is very exciting. Collectively it is beginning to unravel the mysteries of how memories are formed, how memories are stored, and how memory can be improved.

The FDA and Nootropics

The Food and Drug Administration (FDA) is primarily disease/cure-oriented. Therefore, they are not likely to approve new drugs for prevention of degenerative diseases or drugs that claim to improve people's memories. For this reason drug companies are forced to stay with a very traditional disease-oriented approach in the development and marketing of these new drugs. Some of the drug companies are focusing on Alzheimer's disease, which is characterized by impaired memory and cognitive functions.

In its most benign form, Alzheimer's may cause forgetfulness or momentary lapses in recall. In its most severe form the disease may result in brain deterioration to the point where victims are mentally incompetent and helpless. With the aging of our national population, the treatment of cognitive disorders in the elderly is of increasing importance. Approximately 5 percent of the population at age sixty-five is affected and up to 20 percent of the population over eighty years of age is affected. A drug that is even somewhat effective in treating the debilitating memory loss associated with Alzheimer's disease would satisfy the FDA's regulatory requirements, and it would most likely find immediate acceptance in the marketplace.

Another therapeutic area that some drug companies are targeting for their entry into the nootropic race is in the treatment of patients with multiple-infarct dementia. This is a brain disorder that develops as the result of a series of small strokes. It affects an estimated two hundred thousand people in the United States each year. Nootropic drugs hold great promise in helping to restore at least part of the lost memory, and enable victims of this kind of dementia to use the remaining brain capacity to its fullest extent.

When these new memory-enhancing drugs become available in the United States, they will be marketed in association with a disease. The health and memory-enhancing benefits of these drugs will still be the same as is reported in this book, but the drugs will not be advertised or marketed for these unique uses. I urge all of you to read Appendix A, which is an actual FDA Drug Bulletin. In this bulletin the FDA encourages physicians to use approved drugs for "unapproved" uses. The department is telling physicians that this is not only legal, but is one of the primary means of therapeutic innovation. You may need to have your doctor read sections of this book when you tell him/her what it is you want and why you want it.

Possible Mechanisms of Action

It is still not clear how nootropic drugs act to enhance cognitive processes, particularly learning. The fact that most of an ingested nootropic drug will be excreted in the urine unchanged is especially puzzling. The most recent theory suggests that a combination of effects may be involved. Nootropic drugs may:

1. Increase the energy available to the brain cell.
2. Enhance the uptake of choline into the cell.
3. Increase the firing rate of individual cells.

Drug Companies Developing Nootropics

Several major drug companies are currently developing nootropic drugs. A brief discussion of these companies and their
specific versions of a nootropic drug follows.

Syntex Laboratories, Inc. Syntex is the U.S. distributor of
piracetam. Syntex reportedly hopes to have FDA approval for
piracetam by 1989. Piracetam has already proven enormously
successful on a worldwide basis. Syntex is hoping that piracetam will be the first nootropic drug approved by the FDA in the
United States. There will be a significant advantage to the first
approved and available nootropic to hit the market. Because
piracetam is the first discovered and most widely researched
nootropic drug, it will be covered in depth in the next chapter.

Ayerst Laboratories. Ayerst is a division of American Home
Products Corp. Vinpocetine is the name of their entry in the race
to develop a memory-enhancing drug. Vinpocetine was discovered in the 1970s by chemists in Budapest, Hungary. It is
currently available throughout much of Eastern Europe, Mexico, Central America, and Japan. Vinpocetine is a synthetic
chemical that is closely related to the active compounds in
periwinkle, a common garden plant.

Ayerst has carried out animal experiments to test the effectiveness of vinpocetine. A series of tests, designed to measure
memory in laboratory rats, uses a two-chambered box. One
chamber is lit and the other remains dark. Normally rats will
instinctively want to enter the dark chamber, but they can be
easily taught to enter the lit chamber. Exposing the rats to either
scopolamine (a memory-inhibiting drug) or decreased oxygen

(hypoxia) causes them to forget that they were trained to enter the lit chamber. Vinpocetine quickly restored their memory for this task.

To test long-term memory, the rats were taught to enter the lit chamber and then retested three days later. After three days, only about 15 percent of the rats remembered the task. However, 75 percent of the rats treated with vinpocetine correctly remembered the task. Ayerst scientists report that in animal models vinpocetine:

1. Speeds up the rate of learning in laboratory animals by about 40 percent.
2. Helps the animals retain memories for longer periods of time.
3. Blocks the action of drugs that disrupt memory.[3]

Clinical trials with vinpocetine are focusing on the treatment of multiple-infarct dementia. In a trial with human volunteers 67 percent of the people showed significant improvement. A long-term clinical trial with 288 patients lasted over six months. Significant improvement was seen in 77 percent of the vinpocetine-treated patients.[4] Results from both animal and human trials seem to indicate that vinpocetine has definite cognitive-activating ability.

In human trials vinpocetine improved memory and recall. In patients with cerebrovascular disorders, vinpocetine improved both immediate and delayed word recall.[5] In another test normal volunteers using vinpocetine registered improved performance on a test that is specifically designed to test short-term memory (The Sternberg Memory Scanning Task).[6]

Although vinpocetine's mechanism of action is not understood completely, some of its beneficial effects are thought to be the result of its ability to increase cerebral blood flow and improve the glucose fuel uptake in brain cells.[7]

Tests with vinpocetine indicate that it is active in a broad range of pathological conditions that compromise memory functions. These therapeutic applications make it a good candidate for FDA new-drug approval. The fact that it also exhibits significant beneficial effects on healthy humans ensures that it will be one of the top attention-getters as soon as it is marketed.

Hoffmann-La Roche. The maker of Valium and the largest drug company in the world, Hoffmann-La Roche, is making a major commitment to the development of a nootropic compound. Their entry, named aniracetam, is chemically related to piracetam. Early tests with laboratory animals show that aniracetam has remarkable effects in improving and/or normalizing impaired cognitive functions.[8] These results suggest that aniracetam will also be of therapeutic value in humans suffering from impaired cognitive functioning. In comparison with piracetam, aniracetam seems to be active in a broader range of conditions in both improving and protecting memory.[9] In one study of patients with impaired learning and memory, aniracetam proved to be about ten times more potent than piracetam in six out of nine tests used.[10]

In another human trial, sixty patients at a geriatric and nursing home were treated with aniracetam. The study measured the revitalization and resocialization of the patients as reported by the physicians and the staff. The improvements were meaningful and the evaluations by the physicians and the nursing staff showed a high level of agreement. Hoffmann-La Roche expects to initially market aniracetam for cerebrovascular insufficiency.

Warner-Lambert/Parke Davis. Pramiracetam is another variation of the first-known nootropic drug, piracetam. The history of Parke Davis's efforts to find a suitable nootropic drug of their own to develop gives an indication of how important drug companies feel this area is. Researchers at Parke Davis tried 878 other variations of piracetam before they found one with significant cognitive-activating activity. Pramiracetam was the 879th drug tested. Tests with pramiracetam indicate that it enhances several types of learning and long-term memory.[11] Researchers have been able to demonstrate therapeutic effectiveness in three different areas:

1. Learned behavior
2. Improvements in the brain's electrical activity
3. Improvements in the firing rates of individual neurons in the area of the brain known as the hippocampus[12]

Because the hippocampus is involved in working memory and in the process that forms long-term memories, increasing the effectiveness of this area of the brain can help a great deal in improving memory.

The elderly constitute one of the major portions of the population that would use a nootropic drug. Early indications are that this type of therapy would be administered indefinitely, and therefore the safety of pramiracetam and the other nootropics is of increasing interest. As a class of drugs, the cognitive activators or nootropics are essentially entirely free of toxic effects, even at doses far in excess of those required for the therapeutic effects.[13] Pramiracetam has been shown to be very safe in human trials. This allows researchers to continue their efforts for a more accurate understanding of the drug's effects on cognition. Pramiracetam does not interact directly with any known neurotransmitter system and the mechanism by which it activates cognition is not yet known.

Pramiracetam may be an effective treatment for the memory loss experienced by some of the seven hundred thousand Americans who suffer head injuries every year. Pramiracetam may also be useful as a treatment for children with dyslexia.[14]

In a research report to clients, a major investment firm called pramiracetam "the most intriguing new drug at Warner-Lambert/Parke Davis." The reason behind the firm's interest was pramiracetam's unusually positive results in early human trials on patients with Alzheimer's disease. Patients receiving pramiracetam became active and improved to the point that they could recognize immediate family members and could resume

goal-oriented tasks such as cooking and dressing for themselves. Regaining the motivation and ability to perform even a
seemingly commonplace activity is a tremendous accomplish-
ment for an Alzheimer's victim.

Ciba-Geigy. Oxiracetam is a nootropic drug that is reportedly
two to three times more potent than piracetam.[15] In animals, it
has been shown to be very effective at increasing the rate of
learning, increasing the ability to fix new memories, and
memory retention.[16]

Oxiracetam and piracetam were compared in a number of
animal studies exploring learning and memory. They were
essentially equal in several tests. However, oxiracetam showed
distinctly improved results in tests of memory retention and
acquisition.[17]

Investigations designed to discover oxiracetam's mechanism
of action suggest that it activates nerve pathways in the cerebral
cortex and hippocampal areas of the brain.

In one study researchers compared the activity and tolerabil-
ity of oxiracetam with piracetam in the treatment of elderly
patients with the clinical symptoms typical of cerebrovascular
insufficiency (i.e., alterations in intellectual performance, behavior, and psychomotor activity). Both drugs produced favorable effects on psychosomatic and neurologic symptoms, but
oxiracetam produced superior therapeutic results. In particular,
oxiracetam was more effective in relieving mental symptoms
such as impairment of memory, confusion, impaired alertness,
anxiety, and depression. Oxiracetam, like the other nootropics,
is extremely well tolerated and virtually without side effects.

The therapeutic effectiveness of oxiracetam during long-term
treatment also needs to be highlighted. It shows the ability to
produce progressive improvement in clinical symptoms, which
indicates that its effectiveness may actually increase as treatment is continued. This suggests that prolonged treatment may
be more effective.[18]

Another fascinating property of oxiracetam has been re-searched and reported. Female laboratory mice were given oxiracetam throughout their pregnancy. After the prenatally exposed mice were born, they were allowed to grow to maturity and were then tested as adults. The adult mice that were exposed to oxiracetam prenatally showed improved memory capability when compared with untreated mice.[19] The authors of the study point out that, from this study alone, it is inappropriate to suggest that prenatal administration of oxirace-tam (or nootropic drugs in general) can improve the learning ability of adult animals. There is the possibility that what was discovered in this study is specific to the one type of memory capability tested. However, one must admit that this piece of research is certainly interesting and raises many new questions. The fact that administration of a cognitive activating drug to a pregnant mouse can show long-lasting positive effects on the offspring opens up another fascinating area that begs for further research.

Although there are obvious similarities between oxiracetam and piracetam, there are enough differences in their behavioral effects to suggest that they may have different modes or sites of activity.

A similar situation exists in comparing others of the nootro-pic analogs to the first-discovered piracetam. The search for an understanding of the similarities and differences in this fascinating class of drugs will probably make a substantial contribution to our understanding of the physiological and biochemical basis of memory processing.

Progress Report

I recently spoke with research scientists at several of the major drug companies. I learned that the research leading up to FDA licensing approval is going slower than planned. It will proba-bly be several years yet before the nootropics start to be approved in the United States. The problem centers around several issues.

First, to satisfy FDA protocol, researchers have to target a disease for which the drug is useful. A drug that simply enhances or promotes wellness does not fit within the guidelines of the FDA. Senility and Alzheimer's disease seem to be the most appropriate diseases for treatment with nootropic drugs. However, due to the nature of Alzheimer's disease, researchers have been unable to develop an appropriate animal model as a yardstick to test and measure effectiveness of nootropics.

Second, researchers are unable to determine exactly how nootropic drugs exert their effects. The FDA does not usually extend approval to a new drug without an explanation and understanding of how and why it works.

Third, there is no evidence of toxicity associated with nootropic drugs even with extremely large dosages. Frustrated by the inability to establish toxicity, a drug company executive recently told me that a person could eat an entire room full of nootropic drugs and not show any signs of toxicity. Without the ability to measure toxicity, it is difficult to establish dosage ranges. Also, toxicity is a means of evaluating where, how, and why a drug works.

Final Comments

Nootropic drugs present fascinating and amazing potential in the field of memory enhancement. Pharmaceutical companies continue to commit enormous amounts of their time and money to the research and development of these drugs.

Dr. B. P. H. Poschel of Warner-Lambert/Parke Davis has recently written about the new pharmacologic perspectives on nootropic drugs. He stated,

Still, nootropic drugs offer real future promise. That they act somehow in the brain to promote and speed learning in animals appears incontestable. Moreover, since these drugs are essentially entirely free of side effects, even at enormous doses, their use in weakened and aged patients becomes extremely attractive. . . . It is also likely that the ultimate drug of this class has not yet been discovered and/or proven in clinical trials.[20]

Those of us who are interested in health, the prevention of aging, and optimally functioning brains and minds will be anxiously watching the worldwide development and study of this class of drugs.

14

Piracetam: A Drug for the Mind

Piracetam is a cerebral stimulant that appears to act on the cerebral cortex and related structures without any of the side effects normally produced by other cerebral stimulants. Since the cerebral cortex is the site of the brain activity that is associated with human thought and reasoning, any drug that improves its function is extremely important.

Piracetam seems to affect selectively the anterior part of the forebrain. The forebrain is the upper part of the brain, including the cerebral hemispheres. In comparing the human brain with the brain of other creatures, it is the forebrain that shows extraordinary development in size and functional capabilities. The evolutionary inheritance of a massive forebrain is what allows man to be on the leading edge of evolution.

Effects

Piracetam has a number of distinct effects:

1. It protects the brain against damage from oxygen starvation (hypoxia) and also enhances brain recovery from such an event.
2. It increases the rate of metabolism and energy level of brain cells.
3. It enhances learning and memory in healthy volunteers as well as in people who are memory impaired.

4. It protects against memory loss from physical injury and chemical poisoning.

5. It facilitates the transfer of information between the two halves of the brain. This is called interhemispheric flow of information.

Learning and Memory Facilitation

Piracetam has been tested on both animals and humans. In all cases, animals that receive piracetam learn more quickly and better than animals that receive a placebo. One study investigates the ability of rats to learn to avoid a small shock.[1] A much higher percentage of piracetam-treated rats learn to avoid the site of the shock than rats in the control group.

Several studies with human volunteers have demonstrated piracetam's positive effects on mental performance. Dimond and Browers (1976) found that, after two weeks a group of students who received piracetam (4.8 gm/day) had a significant improvement in memory for verbal material compared to a control group.[2]

This study was confirmed in a similar study of seventeen young, healthy volunteers with the administration of 3.2 gm of piracetam per day for five days.[3] Mindus and associates studied eighteen middle-aged subjects who were essentially in good mental health, but complained of some memory loss. The authors reported that piracetam produced significant improvement in mental performance after four weeks of doses of 4.8 gm/day.[4]

Studies of piracetam with both animals and humans are exciting because they show improvement in mental performance in both young and aged subjects.

"Superconnecting" Both Halves of the Brain

Man seems to be the only animal species that has a clear-cut difference between the functions of the two halves of the brain.

Therefore, the flow of information between the two brain hemispheres is essential for harmonious and optimal mental activity. Piracetam actually increases the flow of information between the two halves of the brain.

The two brain hemispheres are connected with a cable-like bundle of nerve fibers called the *corpus callosum*. It is mainly through these fibers that impulses from one hemisphere are transmitted to the other.

One way to test the connection between the two halves of the brain is by teaching rats to avoid shocks through visual stimuli. Each eye sends its information mainly to the opposite side of the brain. If the rats are trained with one eye covered then the opposite half of the brain receives most of the visual information and the primary memory trace (called an engram) will be recorded there.

The other hemisphere will also be informed, but only indirectly, via *corpus callosum* communication. It forms what is called a secondary engram. A secondary engram is always weaker than the primary one. The difference can be measured with memory retention tests. Studies by Buresova and Bures showed that piracetam facilitates the callosal "writing-in" mechanism of the secondary engram.[5]

Human Data

There is a similar test of communication between the brain's hemispheres involving hearing. The subject wears earphones and different words are transmitted simultaneously into each ear. A normal right-handed individual will usually recall more of the words that were presented to the right ear than to the left ear. This is probably due to the existence of a "speech center" which, in right-handed people, is located in the left hemisphere of the brain (see Figure 5).

The nerves from the ears cross over to the opposite side of the brain as do the nerves from the eyes. Therefore, words received

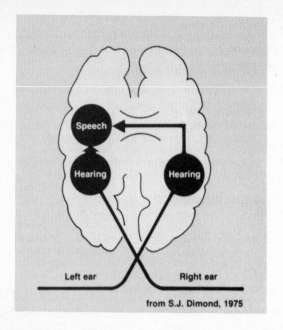

from S.J. Dimond, 1975

FIGURE 5. Direct and crossed pathways reaching the "speech center"—information received by the right ear directly reaches the speech center while that coming from the left ear needs a supplementary pathway.

by the right ear directly reach the left speech center. Those coming from the left ear have to reach the right hearing center first and then are transmitted via the *corpus callosum* to the left speech center.[6]

In the test, information presented to the left ear is sent to the hearing center on the right side of the brain. In order to be understood, the information from the right side's hearing center must be transferred by the *corpus callosum* to the speech center on the left side of the brain.

In this experiment Dr. Dimond tested verbal memory in healthy young volunteers using piracetam. These tests showed that verbal memory is significantly improved with piracetam. A large part of the memory enhancement is due to an increase in the response to information presented to the left ear.[7] This experiment showed that piracetam increases the interhemispheric flow of information. Dr. Dimond concluded that with piracetam, the brain seems to be "*superconnected.*"

Piracetam Increases Brain Energy

Cellular energy production depends upon the systematic build-up and breakdown of a compound called adenosine triphosphate (ATP).[8] Biological aging decreases the amount of ATP available for conversion into energy, particularly in brain and muscle cells. This, in turn, weakens the enzyme-induced processes that trigger the release of energy within the cells. Thus, as most people grow older, they find it increasingly difficult to perform under mental and physical stress, especially for long periods of time.

Piracetam seems to act on the cerebral cortex of the brain to stimulate the production of ATP within cells, and this facilitates transfer of information between the two cerebral hemispheres (ATP is the major energy-producing chemical in the cell). One study that supports this hypothesis showed that piracetam increased the activity of the enzyme that produces ATP.[9] This process may be responsible for piracetam's ability to improve learning capacity.[10]

[CO-ENZYME Q10 ?

Increased Protein Synthesis

Some scientists believe the learning process involves synthesizing new proteins that become part of the structure of brain cells as new information is stored in memory. Piracetam produces major improvements in animal learning. This may be due to the fact that it increases protein synthesis in the brain.

Studies from several laboratories have shown that piracetam has the unique ability to increase the synthesis of proteins in brain cells. It stimulates special cell structures, called polyribosomes, to manufacture these new proteins. The administration of piracetam for short periods of time produced a substantial increase in these special protein-manufacturing structures.[11] It is well established that the storage of long-term memory is dependent on the synthesis of protein in the brain cells.

Piracetam and Dyslexia

In the last several years several reports have been published suggesting that piracetam may be of use in treating children with learning difficulties because of its ability to improve selectively the efficiency of higher cognitive functions. These early studies suggested that dyslexics treated with piracetam have shown improvements in reading skills, verbal memory and verbal conceptualizing ability, feature analysis, and processing of letter-like stimuli. A recent study published in 1987 is titled, "Piracetam and Dyslexia: Effects on Reading Tests."

This study was conducted with two hundred dyslexic children between the ages of seven years six months to twelve years eleven months. The study was of thirty-six-week duration and a double-blind study design. The results of the study showed that the piracetam-treated dyslexics increased their reading fluency without sacrificing accuracy, and those with poor short-term memory increased their digit span scores.[12]

A number of special studies were conducted within the larger study. Researchers conducting one part of the study reported that dyslexics treated in double-blind fashion with piracetam increased their verbal memory, reduced the amount forgotten on a delayed recall trial, and also recorded marked improvement on a special reading test. The results were not only significant statistically, but also showed a meaningful overall gain of six months on reading scores conducted within this twelve-week period.[13]

Another group reported the results of a twelve-week study and found that in this relatively short treatment period, piracetam enhanced the verbal conceptualizing ability (similarities) but did not influence vocabulary as shown by work definitions.

Chase and co-workers reported a marked improvement in reading speed and writing accuracy in dyslexics. This group also analyzed their data to determine the effect of speed upon accuracy and comprehension of reading. The interesting result was that the placebo group had to slow down their reading to improve accuracy; the piracetam-treated dyslexics were able to increase both speed and accuracy at the same time.[14]

Conners and associates reported significant piracetam effects from their study that led them to conclude that "piracetam may increase the efficiency of a left-hemisphere cortical processor intimately involved in letter recognition."[15]

These improvements were evident over a thirty-six-week period, which is one of the longest controlled trials of its kind. In all cases, the medication was well tolerated with no significant side effects reported. This work suggests important possible advancements in the treatment of the many children that fight with lifelong learning disability and the frustrations of dyslexia.

New Developments

Another possible effect of piracetam deserves mention. Research previously mentioned has shown that piracetam facilitates the flow of information between the left and right hemisphere and "superconnects" the brain. This superconnection improves some aspects of the brain's information-handling ability and may increase intelligence.

Some scientists are beginning to speculate about other possible effects of piracetam that may prove to be more exciting and far-reaching in their implications. Integrating communication between the left and right hemispheres of the brain may produce increases in insightfulness and creativity. Piracetam may allow us to integrate the thinking of our rational, conscious mind while receiving information from our intuitive, subconscious mind. It has been proposed that this simultaneous information processing is the source of the creativity and sudden insights that great scientists and artists have.

Classification

Piracetam is the first compound in a completely new class of psychoactive drugs. The word nootropic (Gr.: *noos* = mind; *tropein* = toward) has been coined by Dr. C. Giurgea for this new class of drugs. Nootropics are cerebral stimulants that directly improve particular functions of the forebrain.[16]

Side Effects

Virtually all drugs (both legal and illegal) that act on the central nervous system produce undesirable side effects in addition to the sought-after benefits. One rarely finds a drug that selectively improves mental capabilities, such as the ability to learn and recall, without some accompanying undesirable side effects. Piracetam is a very special and important new drug because it is the first of a long-sought-after class of drugs that does produce important mental benefits without the accompanying side effects. This is why piracetam necessitated the creation of an entirely new class of drugs, the Nootropics.

Even at very high dosage levels piracetam does not produce the side effects that accompany the use of other drugs that affect the central nervous system (such as amphetamines, cocaine, Ritalin, etc.). A review that summarizes over thirty scientific experiments on piracetam, conducted in several animal species, has shown that large doses of piracetam do not

1. Produce sedation or tranquilization. Also, there is no interference with connections between brain cells.
2. Produce changes in brain wave function. Such changes are a major side effect of most drugs that stimulate the central nervous system.

3. Have negative effects on the circulatory, respiratory, or digestive systems.[17]

Toxicity

The toxicity of piracetam has been extensively tested for large single doses (acute toxicity) and long-term use (chronic toxicity). These studies have concluded uniformly that piracetam is nontoxic.[18]

Acute Toxicity: In testing acute toxicity, no toxic symptoms were observed following intravenous doses of up to 8 gm/km to rats, mice, and dogs. For purposes of comparison, a 170 pound human would have to take 618 gm (1.34 pounds)!

Chronic Toxicity: No symptoms of toxicity have been observed after giving rats and dogs large doses for up to a year.

Human Toxicity: No toxic symptoms have been recorded following administration of the drug to humans.

Contraindications

Piracetam has no known contraindications and it has a wide range of safety. Beneficial effects are obtained in relatively small doses, yet large doses (a thousand times greater) are safe and without toxicity or side effects.

How Supplied

Piracetam is marketed by several drug companies, each with its own brand name. The following list, although probably not complete, is a summary of the information found in the literature during the process of researching this book.

TRADE NAME	DRUG COMPANY	WHERE MARKETED
Nootropil	UBC Laboratories	Belgium
		South Africa
		Mexico
Nootropyl	Ucepha	France

Normabrain	Cassella-Ridel	Germany
Dinagen	Hormona Labs	Mexico

I have only been able to obtain samples of the brands of piracetam from Mexico for product identification. Both Nootropil and Dinagen are two-colored, yellow/orange capsules; each capsule contains 400 mg of piracetam. They are packaged and sold in bottles containing sixty capsules per bottle. Dinagen is also marketed as a 400 mg foil-wrapped tablet, with sixty tablets per box.

Dosage Range

In reviewing the literature, three dosage levels have been most frequently used in human trials.

DIRECTIONS	TOTAL DAILY DOSAGE
2 capsules (800 mg) twice daily	1.6 gm
2 capsules (800 mg) three times daily	2.4 gm
4 capsules (1.6 gm) three times daily	4.8 gm

How to Obtain Piracetam

Piracetam is not available in the United States. However, it is available in Mexico and throughout Europe. Piracetam may also be available from the following mail order source: Pharmaceuticals International (see Appendix B).

The situation with piracetam is much the same as that of Lucidril. They are both safe, nontoxic and very beneficial. Unfortunately, they have not been approved by the FDA for use in the United States. Although piracetam is not currently available in the U.S., there is encouraging news to report. Several American pharmaceutical companies are currently testing analogs of piracetam that show considerable promise as memory-enhancing drugs.[19]

Cost of Piracetam

I am not familiar with the prices in Europe. The current price for Dinagen and Nootropil in Mexico, as of this writing (October 1988), is approximately U.S. $6.00 per bottle of sixty capsules.

Final Comments

Piracetam and the other nootropic drugs being developed are exciting for a number of reasons. They have great potential as intelligence-enhancing drugs and, as we try to learn more about how they function, we are learning more about how the brain and memory work.

The next chapter will discuss the results from one of the first attempts at using combinations of intelligence drugs. The combination of the nutrient choline and the drug piracetam may be the most potent memory-enhancing therapy yet discovered.

MY NOTE:

PIRACETAM MAY POTENCIAT THE EFFECTIVENESS OF SUBLIMINAL MESSAGES THROUGH ITS "SUPERCONECTING" EFFECT! (LEFT EAR SUBLIMINAL) (RIGHT EAR AUDIBLE)

15

Piracetam + Choline: A Memory-Enhancing Combination

Usually when we take two or more drugs at the same time, we have to be on the lookout for possible damaging interactions. But there are exceptions to this rule. Exciting results from recent studies have shown that the combination of the nutrient choline and the drug piracetam may be the most potent memory-enhancing therapy yet discovered.

The first report on this research was an animal study published in the March 1981 issue of *The Neurobiology of Aging*.[1] The results of a study with human subjects was published by the same authors in the June 11, 1981, issue of *The New England Journal of Medicine*.[2]

The October 1982 issue of *Anti-Aging News* reviewed these two research projects.[3] In addition, the author did an excellent job of presenting some of the important aspects of the relationship between aging and the gradual decline of mental capabilities. Much of the information in this chapter is drawn from the three sources just mentioned.

Senility and the Aging Brain

Most people under the age of forty never think about senility. That's unfortunate, because the biological aging of the brain is a gradual, progressive process and the symptoms usually are not noticeable until later in life. To optimize mental functioning and minimize the aging of the brain, preventive measures must be taken throughout life. When the symptoms of senility do begin to appear, a lot of damage has already occurred. Advancing senility can be stopped and some of the damage can be reversed. But, nothing beats prevention!

The most dramatic examples of memory loss associated with aging are seen in the elderly who are diagnosed as senile. This condition is characterized by actual damage to brain cells. These brain lesions seriously interfere with the ability of brain cells to communicate with each other. The result is impaired learning capacity and reduced thinking and recall capabilities.

Senile individuals frequently are unable to think clearly. They may find it difficult to remember recent events, they may be confused easily, and they often become incapacitated in stressful situations. As the disease progresses, senile patients are less and less able to take care of their own personal needs (dressing, eating, bathing, and going to the toilet).

Scientists from several different disciplines have been able to demonstrate that most people suffer from some degree of brain damage as they grow older. This gradual process is the result of biological aging; however, much of it can be prevented by proper nutrition and healthy life style habits.

Examination of brains from recently deceased elderly individuals, who were *NOT* yet suffering from senility, have shown a significant loss of dendrites (the delicate hair-like branches of neurons that receive messages from other neurons). This point emphasizes the fact that even though the symptoms of senility are not apparent outwardly, the damage is accumulating in the brain.

The first signs and symptoms of senility do not indicate the beginning of the disease, they indicate the end. The same is true with cancer; a tumor is not the beginning of the disease, it is the end. Currently, chronic degenerative diseases kill far more people than infectious diseases ever did in the past, and most of them are preventable.

We must pay attention to health long before the onset of disease. Extensive internal damage can occur before the actual disease is noticeable. For example, when the first signs and symptoms of high blood pressure appear, the arteries already may have lost over 50 percent of their volume to plaque buildup, and frequently the first sign of heart disease is death.

Many drugs that are used to treat age-associated disorders have been shown to be effective in increasing mental performance, improving stamina and coordination, and extending lifespan in normally aging animals. There is encouraging evidence that these drugs also help humans in similar ways.

Choline and Piracetam

Now there is exciting new evidence that a combination of the nutrient choline and the drug piracetam may be far more effective in treating the mental decline of aging than either substance alone.

Efforts to improve mental functioning by administering choline produced inconsistent results. Dr. Raymond Bartus, formerly of the American Cyanamid Corporation, had the idea of combining choline and piracetam to treat age-related memory loss. Dr. Bartus speculated that one reason for the failure of some choline studies might be that the aged brain is unable to transform extra amounts of choline into acetylcholine.

Dr. Bartus then hypothesized that it might be necessary to improve other factors to produce the desired mental benefits from dietary choline in the elderly. One such factor, brain energy metabolism, has been shown to decline with advancing age.

Energy production in the brain appears to be essential for effective information processing. Therefore, Bartus thought that the effect of supplemental choline or lecithin might be enhanced by the use of an agent to improve brain energy metabolism. This line of reasoning led him to piracetam.

Piracetam has been shown to improve several mental abilities in humans. Evidence suggests that it may act by stimulating the activity of ATP (adenosine triphosphate) in brain cells. Since ATP is the primary source of energy in brain cells, Bartus thought that it might help to improve the ability of brain cells to transform dietary choline into acetylcholine, and thereby improve thinking ability in older individuals.

Assessing Memory Function

Dr. Bartus designed a study to test his hypothesis using aged laboratory rats (twenty-three to twenty-nine months of age). He set up an experiment to assess memory function. The apparatus for this test is a two-chamber box. One chamber is open at the top (i.e., illuminated) and the second chamber is enclosed (i.e., dark). Lab technicians control a sliding door between the two compartments.

Each rat was placed in the illuminated chamber with the door between the illuminated and dark chambers closed. Rats always prefer a dark area if they have a choice. After a three-second orientation period, the door was raised, allowing the rat to freely explore the apparatus. As soon as it discovers and enters the dark chamber, a technician closes the door. An electric shock (harmless but unpleasant) is then delivered to the animal through the floor grid for three seconds. Following this unpleasant experience, the rat was returned to its home cage to await retention testing.

Twenty-four hours later, each rat was returned to the chamber-box. The length of time a rat avoids reentering the dark chamber (the source of the electrical shock) is a measure of the animal's memory retention of the previously administered shock.

Extensive testing has shown that rats find it increasingly

difficult to remember such an experience as they grow older. The performance of aged rats is comparable to that of young rats when tested within an hour after training. However, the memory in aged rats decreases sharply if they are tested several hours later. Testing aged rats for memory retention twenty-four hours after training shows that there are substantial losses in memory. These findings suggest that rats suffer serious memory losses due to aging and that these losses are comparable to those observed in humans as well as other species of test animals.

Four separate groups of animals were tested in this particular study. One group was the control group, the second was the choline group, the third was the piracetam group, and the fourth group of animals was tested with the combination of choline + piracetam.

Results of the Study

The animal's memory is determined by how long it takes the rat to enter the dark chamber during the Test Performance. This is a measure of how well the animal retained the memory of the electrical shock it received through the floor of the dark chamber during the pre-training performance twenty-four hours earlier. Previous research has shown that rats of this age (twenty-three to twenty-nine months) suffer a severe impairment of short-term memory retention from the electric shock in this type of test.

There were no significant differences in the pre-training performance of all four groups of rats. However, when the animals were retested twenty-four hours later, significant differences in performance were noted. The rats given choline scored slightly better than the control group (not statistically significant). The rats in the piracetam group showed a small but statistically reliable improvement on retention scores over the control group, scoring slightly better than the choline group.

Results

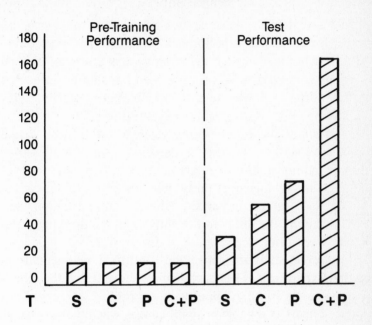

T = time seconds
S = rats receiving saline injections as controls
C = rats receiving choline
P = rats receiving piracetam
C + P = rats receiving combination of choline + piracetam

FIGURE 6. Effects of Saline, Choline, Piracetam, or Choline + Piracetam on a Twenty-Four-Hour Passive Avoidance Memory Retention Test

However, as seen in Figure 6, the rats given the combination of choline plus piracetam showed dramatically higher memory retention scores. They scored about four times higher than the control group and about three times higher than the animals given piracetam alone.[4]

Replication

In order to replicate and extend the findings from the first study, another experiment was performed.[5] Its major purposes were:

1. To determine whether the improvement under the choline piracetam combination was simply due to adding the effects of the two drugs or was due to a multiplying effect. This multiplying effect is also called a synergistic effect.

2. To study the difference between a single dose (acute administration) and the use of the drug over a longer time (chronic administration). Acute administration consisted of giving a single injection thirty minutes prior to the initial training and test performances. Chronic administration consisted of giving the drugs to the animals in the drinking water for one week prior to testing.

This second study replicated and confirmed the results from the first experiment. The second study showed that the effects from twice the dose of piracetam or choline alone did not produce effects as reliable or significant as when the two agents were administered simultaneously. Also, the longer the combination was administered, the greater the effects.

The results of these studies indicate that a combination of choline and piracetam can produce major improvements in memory function in rats and that this effect is synergistic.

Choline + Piracetam: Human Clinical Trail

S. H. Ferris and his associates at the New York University School of Medicine, Department of Psychiatry, learned of the impressive results achieved by Dr. Bartus. They decided to explore the effects of combined choline/piracetam therapy in patients suffering from Alzheimer's disease (a common cause of senility). The clinical trial was designed to verify the safety, tolerance, and possible efficacy of combined choline/piracetam therapy. Subjects were treated for seven days with 9 gm of choline and 4.8 gm of piracetam per day, administered in three equally-divided doses.

The results showed small improvements in most cognitive measures for the entire group. However, during the evaluation period, it soon became apparent that 30 percent of the patients were achieving truly *dramatic clinical improvements*—far greater than had ever been observed with either choline or piracetam alone! For example, scores on one test showed a mean improvement of 70 percent in verbal memory retrieval!

After examining the blood chemistries, Dr. Ferris believes there may be a subgroup among patients suffering from Alzheimer's disease that can be helped dramatically by choline/piracetam therapy.[6]

Nootropic Drugs + Choline Supplementation

The powerful synergistic effects of piracetam and choline was an exciting discovery. Recent understanding of how and why this synergistic effect works may make choline a necessary partner to therapy with nootropic drugs. A leading scientist in this field, R. J. Wurtman from MIT, has said that nootropic drugs may be contraindicated in Alzheimer's disease unless concurrent supplemental doses of choline or lecithin are given. An explanation of this follows.

Cholinergic neurons are the brain cells that secrete the neurotransmitter acetylcholine for thought and memory processes. Scientists at MIT have pointed out that cholinergic neurons have two uses for phosphatidyl choline. One is in the structure of their cellular membranes. The other use is inside the cell where the choline from phosphatidyl choline is used to manufacture the neurotransmitter acetylcholine.[7]

When the cholinergic neurons are stimulated, acetylcholine is secreted and the level of choline inside the cell gets depleted. The internal depletion of choline is greatest when the neuron is firing rapidly and/or when the supply of extracellular choline is low.

The MIT scientists believe that the cholinergic neuron is unique in that it can break down its own membrane to obtain the needed choline to make more acetylcholine if the extracellular supply of choline is inadequate. This situation is referred to as "auto-cannibalism" and it can lead to the eventual death of the cell.[8]

Treating Alzheimer's disease with nootropic drugs without choline supplements could increase the firing rate of the neurons in an elderly patient whose diet is low in choline (lecithin). While an initial benefit might be seen in the Alzheimer patient, the long-term effects could be harmful because "auto-cannibalism" might be increased.

A new ideal has also been proposed. Giving a patient with Alzheimer's disease supplemental choline or high-potency lecithin might help to reduce the amount of "auto-cannibalism." Therefore, even if choline/lecithin do not have a rapid and direct effect on Alzheimer symptoms, they may possibly be effective at limiting or retarding the progress of the disease.[9]

One answer often creates new questions. Such is the case with the astounding results obtained by the Bartus and Ferris studies. There is an urgent need for further research. For example, what results will choline/piracetam therapy produce in:

1. Long-term therapy
2. Dosages tailored to the specific needs of individual patients
3. Combination with other nutrients and/or drugs that might be expected to improve cognitive function.

Brain research is a field of study that is still in its infancy, but progress is proceeding at a rapid pace. We can look forward to quantum leaps in our knowledge and understanding of the brain and in our ability to improve its functioning. It is truly a fascinating evolutionary path that we travel.

16

The Herbal Way

Long before recorded history, herbs and herbal preparations provided an excellent natural way to enhance memory, mental alertness, and general mental functioning. Some herbs are also helpful in slowing down the aging process and relieving some of the symptoms of old age.

An herb is a plant that is used for its nutritional value and therapeutic or medicinal properties. Traditionally, herbs have been used in their natural form. Usually the leaves, roots, and bark are powdered or brewed into a tea and ingested or applied to the body.

The earliest written record on the use of herbs was composed five thousand years ago by the Sumerians. A Chinese treatise on herbs dates back to 2700 B.C. and describes 365 herbs and their therapeutic uses.[1] Today, the use of herbs in medicine is widely accepted in Asia, Russia, and some European countries.

Why have herbs largely been ignored or dismissed as "ineffective" by modern Western medicine? The introduction of more specifically potent chemical drugs in the eighteenth and nineteenth centuries led to the dominance of chemical medicine in the twentieth century. The theory of the "active ingredient" was developed to account for the power of herbal treatments. Chemists worked to extract and purify this active ingredient and eliminate the other "unnecessary" components. In this way the strength of the dose could be standardized.

These new preparations were sometimes able to annihilate killer diseases quickly. This resulted in a change in belief system. It was thought that each disease had one cause and could therefore be controlled by a given chemical substance. Inspired by these new, fast, powerful methods of treatment, modern medicine directed its inquiry toward specific diseases and causes, leaving behind the idea of the "whole body" and natural, botanical therapies.

Today we are beginning to realize the value of "ancient wisdom" and see the need for a balance between the natural and the synthetic. We are experiencing a resurgence of interest in "holistic" natural healing and the use of herbal therapies.

The assumption behind natural healing is that the body is capable of healing itself given the proper conditions. Treatment with herbs is not aimed at a given disease. Instead it attempts to energize and stimulate the entire body while supporting the immune system in doing its job.

The herbs we will discuss in this chapter and the chapters on ginseng and ginkgo are known, both in scientific circles and folklore, to stimulate mental activity. There are many active ingredients in individual herbs and herbal blends. Some ingredients are more active for some conditions than others and can have different therapeutic effects in different people.

A particular herb may contain several active ingredients that increase each other's effects. In some herbal blends secondary herbs are added to support the absorption, transport, and effectiveness of the primary herb. Each is integral for the effectiveness of the other.

The level of active ingredients in herbs can vary due to soil conditions, climate, time of year harvested, and method of preparation or extraction. Many products are being prepared now from extracts, which allows for standardization of active ingredients because the strength of a batch can be tested.

Although herbs have therapeutic properties, they should not be thought of or classified as drugs. Herbs contain a mixture of naturally occurring substances that often possess a number of therapeutic effects. Drugs are generally refined, purified, and concentrated forms of a single substance that is designed to have a single therapeutic effect. Herbs are generally more gentle and tonic-like whereas drugs are strong, selective in their effects, and may have toxic side effects.

The scientific documentation, validation, and understanding of herbal therapies has received very little attention in the United States. Pharmaceutical companies find it economically more attractive to develop potent, synthetic, disease-oriented medicines. According to Dan Mowrey, Ph.D., who wrote *The Scientific Validation of Herbal Medicine*, 90 percent of the scientific research on herbs is conducted in Japan, China, the U.S.S.R., and some European countries.[2]

Herbs for Mental Alertness, Memory, and Senility

With the exception of ginseng and *Ginkgo biloba*, scientific data on many of the herbs known by folk and traditional herbal medicine to enhance mental functions is sparse. In my research, I did encounter several blends designed to support brain health and I think they bear mention. One blend found in Dr. Mowrey's book *The Scientific Validation of Herbal Medicine* has detailed information and research on each herb and its function. Because it is so complete and well done, I chose to reprint it in its entirety in this chapter.

Dr. Mowrey states that he has relied on the compilation of hard facts, soft facts, clinical information, cross-cultural verification, and anecdotal clues, with a primary emphasis on hard, scientific information.

Regarding the presentation of the material in the following section, Dr. Mowrey states, "Several herbs are described in each chapter. They may be used separately but it is preferable to blend them together. The major herbs, those with the more potent activity, are listed at the beginning of the chapter in capital letters. The other herbs, though potent in other blends, are meant in this case to augment, modulate or otherwise modify the overall activity of the major herbs. In a blend these interactions would be more strongly felt."

The following is Dr. Mowrey's discussion and formula for his herbal blend.

AN HERBAL BLEND FOR MENTAL ALERTNESS/SENILITY

FORM: Capsule, Tea

CONTENTS: PEPPERMINT (*Mentha piperita*), SIBERIAN GINSENG (*Eleutherococcus senticosus*), skullcap (*Scutellaria lateriflora*), wood betony (*Stachys officinalis*), gotu-kola (*Hydrocotyle asiatica*), and kelp (*Laminaria, Macrocystis, Ascophyllum*).

PURPOSE: To improve poor memory; to increase concentration capability and mental stamina; to overcome the effects of aging on mental attributes.

OTHER APPLICATIONS: Poor circulation, irritability, anxiety, insomnia, hyperactivity, depression.

Use: 1. Adults, general use: As desired, up to 12 capsules per day.
2. Adults, acute conditions: 3–4 capsules, 3 times per day.
3. Hyperactive children: 2–3 capsules in morning; 1–2 capsules at dinner. Use 3–4 capsules of ginger root per day.

CONTRAINDICATIONS: None

With growing age, the blood supply to the brain usually decreases and brings on the death of cerebral neurons. Nerve death is also caused by alcoholism, smoking, vitamin B-complex deficiency, and so on. Decreased mental function invariably results. Similar conditions can result from genetic lesions, biochemical deficits, trauma and maternal prenatal health. Neural cell damage cannot easily be reversed. As a general rule, brain cells do not replace themselves. Sometimes, however, remaining live brain cells can take over the functions of their dead neighbors. Therefore, there is always hope for continued healthy functioning. Mental dysfunction, including poor memory and the inability to concentrate also result from unnecessary restlessness, irritability, hypersensitivity and nervous excitability. The goals of this blend are to help younger, healthy individuals improve the efficiency of their mental faculties, to prevent the onset of senile brain damage, to arrest any degeneration in progress, or delay its onset as long as possible, to help healthy tissue compensate for deficiencies, and secondarily, to curb irritability, hypersensitivity, etc. To accomplish these ends the blend must increase healthy arterial and venous circulation, and improve the general health of the nervous system and the rest of the body, especially the adrenal system. These herbs provide circulation to the cells of the brain, nurture nerves, calm irritability, impart restfulness and clarity of mind, and generally increase mental capabilities. They probably will not reverse any neural damage already sustained, but the increased mental capacity experienced may make you think they have.

Peppermint leaf, due to the presence of several essential oils, prevents congestion of the blood supply to the brain, helps to clear up any circulatory congestion that exists, stimulates circulation, and strengthens and calms nerves. It is this last effect which has been noted so often by clinicians treating deficiencies in the ability to concentrate. The calming effect produced by peppermint allows the patient to apply himself directly to the task at hand. University students have benefited greatly through participation in loosely controlled experiments assessing the effects of peppermint tea on test-taking skills and examination scores.

Siberian Ginseng is, of course, the famous Asiatic tonic, that has been shown in numerous studies to affect mental and physical behavior. In geriatric use, ginseng has been proven beneficial in restoring mental abilities. Ginseng helps by directly affecting the adrenal-pituitary axis, which effect is most often manifested as increased resistance to the effects of stress. The herb also aids mental function by improving circulation. Studies have also demonstrated the ability of ginseng to help learning. Other studies show that ginseng is a direct central nervous system stimulant. All of these effects, and others discussed more fully in chapters on low blood sugar, fatigue and whole body tonic blends, contribute to the pronounced beneficial effects of ginseng on mental health, the prevention of senility, and the remedy of lost mental powers.

Skullcap is one of the best nervines in the plant kingdom. Read about this herb in the chapters on insomnia, nervous tension, nerves and glands, and pain relief. We note here that this herb probably affects mental abilities by removing the nervous tension that often interferes with learning, recall, logical thinking and memory formation. In this regard, it very much resembles a muscle relaxant.

Wood betony is also a good nervine with known hypotensive properties. It is used primarily to reduce nervousness through a mild sedative action.

Gotu-kola, being a naturally excellent neural tonic, slowly builds mental stamina and neural health. It is an excellent treatment for nervous breakdown. In addition, gotu kola, according to Asian and European practice, is an excellent blood purifier, glandular tonic and diuretic. It is used around the world for diseases of the skin, blood and nervous system, for leprosy and syphilis, psoriasis, cervicitis, vaginitis, blisters, and so forth. India is the country in which gotu-kola is perhaps most popular. There the plant has enjoyed a long history of folk use, and like our goldenseal, its potential uses have been well explored. The people of India use the plant specifically to improve memory and longevity.

Kelp is included in this blend to provide nutritional support to the nervous system and heart, in the form of vitamins, minerals and cell salts. In addition, it supplies a hypotensive principle. This property is likely to have a sparing effect on cardiac and neural tissues, i.e., it saves them from unnecessary stress, prolongs their effective lifetime, and increases their efficiency during daily use. Japanese researchers found that laminaria exhibits definite hypotensive and blood cholesterol lowering activity when given to rabbits and humans. This effect is probably due to histamine content or some combination of minerals or other nutrients.[3]

This concludes the presentation of Dr. Mowrey's formula. If you want to make this preparation for yourself, it is recommended that you mix equal parts of each of the ingredients. You can then brew a tea from the resulting mixture or put it into capsules to take orally.

Other Herbal Blends

There are a number of other herbal blends available that are formulated to support mental functioning. Most blends are simply a mixture of pure herbs, but in some cases, herbal blends have been added to nutritional formulas. The following two blends are examples of each type. The first blend is part of a brain formula that also has amino acids, vitamins, and minerals (see Chapter 28 on brain formulas). The herbs are:

Bee Pollen	125 mg
Ginseng	100 mg
Gotu-Kola	100 mg
Myrtlewood	75 mg
Alfalfa	75 mg
Echinacea	75 mg
Peppermint Leaves	60 mg
Fo-Ti	50 mg
Licorice Root	50 mg
Ginger Root	50 mg
Blue Vervain	50 mg
Sarsaparilla Root	50 mg
Cayenne	40 mg
Kelp	35 mg
Wood Betony	15 mg

The second blend is formulated to act as a brain energizer. It contains the following herbs (the proportions are proprietary information): Myrtlewood, Fo-Ti, Ginseng, Gotu-Kola, American Century, Bissy Nut, Alfalfa, Echinacea, Brigham Tea, Cayenne, Oregon Grape, Ginger Root.

We can see that the two above formulations contain the herbs that Dr. Mowrey has described as offering the strongest support for the brain and mental functioning: ginseng, gotu-kola, and peppermint. Ginkgo, another herb in this class, is a new arrival on the American scene. It can be mixed with other herbs in a preparation or taken separately in capsule form. Since our focus here is on these primary herbs, we will not detail the activities of all the support herbs in these blends. These support herbs in general aid in the transport of oxygen, stimulate circulation, assist in digestion and assimilation, aid in detoxification, and provide general nutritional support.

Final Comments

The plant kingdom has supplied us with many important herbs to support our mental functions. Some of these herbs work by increasing the supply of blood and oxygen to our brains. Others work by stimulating our nervous system, by increasing the brain's ability to utilize glucose and produce mental energy, and by serving as free radical scavengers. Still others work by increasing resistance to the effects of stress that often interfere with concentration, logical thinking, learning, and memory.

17

Ginkgo Biloba: A Medicinal Tree

The most ancient species of tree known provides a remarkable new therapeutic substance that improves short-term memory, eases some symptoms of aging, and is effective against a wide variety of brain disorders. Extracts from the leaves of the *Ginkgo biloba* tree are now being used to stimulate cerebral circulation, to improve mental alertness and overall brain functioning. Some scientists are suggesting that research on *Ginkgo biloba* may lead to a whole new class of medicines.

Before we explore its therapeutic capabilities, let's look at the history and properties of this remarkable tree.

Historical Background

Considered a "living fossil," the *Ginkgo biloba* tree is the most primitive tree on the planet. Fossil records show that ginkgo trees were growing on the earth 300 million years ago. It is the sole surviving member of a prehistoric family of trees, and is the only member of its species, genus, family, order, and class. No other living thing has such singular distinction. Individual trees may live as long as one thousand years.

The ginkgo tree nearly became extinct during the last Ice Age. Two thousand years ago it was nearly driven to extinction by the advance of civilization in China. It was saved by Chinese monks who considered it a sacred tree and grew it inside their temples. In addition to its beauty, the ginkgo tree has another unique characteristic. At high temperatures it secretes a sap that acts as a fire retardant. It is thought that this protective quality is one reason why ginkgo trees surround many Buddhist temples throughout China and Japan.

Ginkgo biloba, also called the maiden hair tree, is an ornamental tree with unique and beautifully shaped leaves. The ginkgo leaf has veins fanning out in two distinct halves. Used for centuries in Chinese medicine as a tonic for the brain, the leaf, interestingly, has a similar appearance to the human brain, hence its name, *Ginkgo biloba* (bi-lobal).

Ginkgo trees now line the streets in many cities around the world. Powerful antioxidant compounds in the ginkgo tree are thought to be responsible for the tree's hardiness and ability to thrive in polluted city environments.

Ginkgo and Modern Science

The fruit and leaf of this ancient tree have been used in Chinese medicine for thousands of years. Tea made from the ginkgo leaf is invigorating and has been valued especially by elderly Chinese. Today, in Asia and the continent of Europe, ginkgo extracts are used extensively. Over 1.2 million prescriptions are being dispensed by doctors in Europe per month, specifically for stimulating circulation to the brain. Annual sales are estimated at $500 million! An indication of ginkgo's importance is exhibited by the fact that a large European phytopharmaceutical company (a company that specializes in medicinal plants) has established a twelve-hundred-tree plantation in South Carolina, distributing the extract primarily to Europe.

In recent years there has been a flurry of modern scientific interest in the medicinal properties of the ginkgo leaf. The pharmacological action of ginkgo extract increases the supply of blood and oxygen to the brain and produces beneficial changes in brain chemistry. Reports also show that the ginkgo extracts increase the supply and utilization of glucose, which is the brain's primary source of fuel and energy.

The bulk of medical research on ginkgo's biological and physiological properties has been conducted in Europe. In September 1986, the prestigious French medical journal *La Presse Medicale* devoted its whole issue to the biochemistry, pharmacology, history, and clinical applications of *Ginkgo biloba*. The results tell us how and why ginkgo has proven to be so effective and provides us with many clinical studies.

Active Ingredients

Ginkgo's pharmacological activity is due to its high content of the following substances:

1. Several groups of flavonoids (the medicinal compounds)
2. Terpinoid substances
3. Vitamin C along with several other organic acids
4. Several carotenoids similar to beta-carotene
5. The iron-based form of superoxide dismutase (SOD).

How Ginkgo Works

Ginkgo biloba extract has demonstrated remarkable pharmacological action on the circulatory and nervous system. Its actions include:

1. Increasing the circulation to the brain and extremities by acting as a vasodilator, especially in the medium and small capillaries.
2. Preventing free radical damage to cellular membranes of sensitive tissues such as the brain, nervous system and liver.
3. Protecting nerve tissue from damage due to decreased supply of blood and oxygen (hypoxia).
4. Enhancing the brain's ability to metabolize glucose, its primary source of fuel and energy.
5. Increasing nerve transmission.

6. Helping repair lesions in cellular membranes caused by free radical damage.

Microcirculation

A decreased blood flow to any tissue or area of the body represents a serious problem. The resulting decrease in oxygen supply increases free radical damage to the tissue. The frequency of this problem is increasing due to the high incidence of cardiovascular disease, particularly atherosclerosis or clogged arteries. This problem is even more serious when it causes a decreased blood flow to the brain.

Ginkgo possesses a unique ability that is not exhibited by any other known substance. It specifically enhances circulation to the microcapillaries. The microcapillaries are the blood vessels that are the smallest and furthest away from the heart. In suboptimal conditions, they are the first to be subjected to a decreased amount of blood and oxygen, making them susceptible to free radical damage and aging. Ginkgo actually stimulates the release of a substance that relaxes the microcapillaries thus increasing blood flow.[1] This means that ginkgo may be the most effective remedy known for many of the "side effects" of aging, such as: short-term memory loss, slow thinking and reasoning, dizziness, ringing in the ears, and problems with vertigo or equilibrium.

A long-term ginkgo study with 166 geriatric patients suffering from chronic cerebral insufficiency showed that it helps to improve mental functioning in elderly patients. The study reported that, "The results confirm that *Ginkgo biloba* extract is effective against cerebral disorders due to aging. The difference between control and treatment groups became significant at three months and increased during the following months."[2]

Senile macular degeneration is a disease of the eye caused by poor circulation. A disease frequently seen in the elderly, it is a common cause of blindness for which there is no satisfactory medical treatment. A double-blind trial with a small number of patients showed that *Ginkgo biloba* extract produced a statistically significant improvement in long distance vision. The scientists doing the research theorize that the improvement is related to *Ginkgo biloba* extract's neutralizing effect on free oxygen radicals produced in the eye.[3]

Hypoxia

Poor circulation creates hypoxia (lack of oxygen), resulting in free radical damage to the tissues. A number of scientific reports document ginkgo's ability to protect against this type of damage.[4] It is suggested that the improvement in brain glucose metabolism and the increased blood supply to brain cells may contribute to ginkgo's protection against hypoxia.

Ginkgo's ability to protect against hypoxic effects is not limited to the elderly population. German scientists devised an ingenious method to create hypoxia in healthy subjects without harming them. This hypoxic model produced the effects of cerebral insufficiency similar to that which commonly develops in the elderly.

This test demonstrated that ginkgo was able to protect against the decrease in the rate of nerve impulse conduction produced by hypoxic conditions. The response time of muscles controlled by the brain was significantly greater than in a hypoxic condition. There was also an improvement in the rate of respiration.[5]

Ginkgo has a powerful ability to reduce free radical damage throughout the entire body. It is both the antioxidant properties of ginkgo's active ingredients and its ability to enhance circulation that reduce hypoxia and the resultant free radical damage.

Short-term Memory

Another study showed that *Ginkgo biloba* extract improves short-term memory. This was a well-designed double-blind crossover study in which healthy volunteers were given a single high dose of *Ginkgo biloba* extract, which was five times the normal dose. One hour later a battery of tests were given and the test group showed a significant improvement in short-term memory.[6]

Mental Alertness

Ginkgo affects mental alertness by actually changing the frequency of brain waves. A double-blind study, in which EEG monitors were used on the subjects, showed that ginkgo extract increases brain alpha rhythms. These are the brain wave frequencies associated with mental alertness. The monitors also indicated a decrease in brain theta rhythms, which are the slower brain frequencies associated with a lack of attention and an "unfocused" state of mind.

This study was conducted with elderly subjects who were exhibiting signs of mental deterioration. A significant increase in mental alertness was seen by the third week of the study. Mental alertness continued to increase throughout the remaining three months of the study. The ginkgo volunteers also showed improvement in some of their physical symptoms, whereas the control group did not.[7]

Alzheimer's Disease and Senility

A survey of many studies on ginkgo concerning its pharmacological and psychopharmacological properties, discusses ginkgo's clinical effectiveness in the elderly. The survey states that *Ginkgo biloba* extract seems to be effective in all types of dementia and even in patients suffering from cognitive disorders resulting from depression. The survey concludes that ginkgo is particularly beneficial for people who are just beginning to experience deterioration in their cognitive functions. The extract may delay deterioration and enable these subjects to maintain a normal life and escape institutionalization.[8]

In another study, experimental data suggested that ginkgo may act on a number of major problems seen in patients with Alzheimer's disease and dementia. The study concludes, "From what is already known about *Ginkgo biloba* extract, it appears that it fulfills the conditions laid down by the World Health Organization concerning the development of drugs effective against cerebral aging."[9]

Dosage

Because most of ginkgo's active ingredients are water-soluble, it is active orally, it is easily digested, and its constituents enter the blood stream easily. The half-life of ginkgo is reported to be about three hours. This means that, three hours after taking a product containing ginkgo, only about half of the amount ingested will remain in the body. The rest will have either been metabolized or excreted. From this we infer that taking ginkgo three times daily would probably be optimal to maintain therapeutic blood levels.

Although high doses of ginkgo have shown fast (one hour) improvements in short-term memory, in general ginkgo is a relatively slow-acting substance. Therefore, a standardized dosage is desirable, and a course of therapy to achieve the desired effects often takes from three to six months.

The concentrated powdered extract is the preferred dosage form. This gives a standardized 24 percent concentration of the flavonoids. However, the majority of products available on the market usually contain a lower level of active ingredients.

The ratio of the active ingredients is important to the activity of *Ginkgo biloba* extract. Most of the scientific research on ginkgo has been performed with a 50:1 ratio. This means that processors used fifty pounds of ginkgo leaves to make one pound of extract. Most of the commercial products available in the United States are only an 8:1 ratio of the extract. To compensate for the lower percentage of active ingredients, the

capsules of these products contain 240 milligrams, which leads
to a recommended daily dosage of 1000 milligrams or about
four capsules.

An average dosage of 24 percent *Ginkgo biloba* extract is
from 120 to 160 milligrams per day, taken in divided doses. It
is nontoxic even at excessive levels. No side effects have been
reported in scientific literature even at levels of 600 milligrams
in a single dose. Exceeding the average dosage should be done
only under the care of a health professional. *Ginkgo biloba*
extract is available in tincture, capsules, and tablets. It is also
found in some brain formulas (see Chapter 28).

Final Comments

Ginkgo biloba extract offers effective treatment for people with
signs and symptoms of reduced blood flow of oxygen to the
brain and other extremities. Ginkgo is shown to be helpful for
many of the complaints of the elderly such as loss of memory,
depression, dizziness, and ringing in the ears. *Ginkgo biloba*
extract is beneficial in increasing mental alertness for people of
all ages. The extract may offer a protective action against
Alzheimer's and other forms of dementia. It is the most
effective agent known for increasing circulation into the microcapillaries.

18

Ginseng: Wonder Herb of the Orient

Ginseng, called the "King of Herbs," is an exciting, potent herb that is rapidly gaining in popularity in the West. The first recorded Chinese treatise on medicine states that ginseng serves "to restore the five internal organs, tranquilize the spirit, calm agitation of the mind, allay excitement, and ward off harmful influences . . . The continual use of ginseng makes for long life with light weight of the body." [1]

Ginseng has been used in Chinese medicine for over four thousand years as a miracle cure-all, elixir of life, and a panacea for almost everything. It is still the most widely used medicinal plant in the Orient. Ginseng has been used to treat conditions such as mental fatigue, insomnia, arthritis, tuberculosis, indigestion, high blood pressure, stress related disorders, cancer, and many more.

Does ginseng deserve this reputation? Because of such a long and extensive record as a curative agent, research scientists from the U.S.S.R., Sweden, Korea, China, Japan, Germany, Argentina, and the United States are investigating the efficacy of ginseng's medicinal value. Clinical effects, pharmacological actions, and chemical properties are being examined. The findings of these scientists are consistent with the historical postulates of ancient and modern Chinese herbalists. According to published data, ginseng:

1. Stimulates and improves brain functions, concentration, memory and learning.
2. Protects against stress and fatigue.
3. Quenches free radicals, thus inhibiting the aging process.
4. Reduces harmful cholesterol levels.
5. Improves cerebrovascular circulation.
6. Reduces heart beat.
7. Normalizes blood pressure.
8. Normalizes blood sugar.
9. Increases endocrine activity and thus metabolic functions.
10. Stimulates circulatory system and digestion.
11. Increases resistance to drugs, alcohol, chemotherapy, and toxins in general.
12. Improves athletic performance.
13. Shortens recovery time after exercise or stressful situations.
14. Benefits insomnia and sleep disturbances.
15. Is an immune stimulant.
16. Augments sexual function.
17. Stabilizes and normalizes bodily functions in general.

Does this sound a bit like the elixir that the traveling "medicine man" claims will cure all your ills? Such an impressive list of benefits certainly can stimulate the skeptical mind. However, what is important to understand here is that ginseng is what is known as an "adaptogen," a term coined by Russian scientists.

Adaptogens

An adaptogen is a nontoxic substance that increases an organism's resistance to adverse stress factors of a physical, chemical, and biological origin. Dr. Kurt Donsbach, one of America's foremost nutritionists and health care educators, states,

Unlike synthetic drugs designed to act against specific disease conditions, Ginseng works in a nonspecific manner and thus is a valuable agent in a broad spectrum of chemical disorders. It sets up a universal defense system capable of increasing the body's resistance to physical factors such as overheating and radiation, to chemical factors such as poisons and cancer-inducing substances, and to biological factors such as bacteria and viruses.

Adaptogens have a remarkable normalizing homeostatic ability, that is, they return the body to normal healthy condition no matter what pathological changes are occurring in the body previous to the administration of the adaptogen.[2]

Ginseng and Mental Functions

What does this mean for those of us seeking to enhance our mental functions? Ginseng is able to modulate physical and mental stresses that inhibit optimal mental functioning and performance.

Research has documented ginseng's ability to improve mental performance of people under stress. Stress and overwork deplete norepinephrine, resulting in mental fatigue and loss of concentration. Norepinephrine is an important brain chemical that effects mind, mood, and memory. Ginseng increases norepinephrine levels when the body is under stress.[3]

There have been many studies that indicate that ginseng will also improve the mental performance of healthy people. One such study was conducted by the Pharmacological Committee of the U.S.S.R. Ministry of Health. They tested a group of telegraph operators, where concentration, coordination, and physical endurance are required. After taking ginseng for thirty days, they showed finer coordination of mental and physical reflexes and increased endurance. The workers made fewer mistakes and demonstrated better concentration.[4]

Blood sugar levels also affect mental functioning. Low blood sugar (hypoglycemia) creates mental fatigue, muddled thinking, and the inability to concentrate. Ginseng normalizes this condition. The exciting thing is that ginseng will also lower blood sugar in people with excessive blood glucose.[5] This shows the power and flexibility of ginseng working in the truest sense as an adaptogen.

A decrease in blood circulation to the brain decreases mental performance. This is most commonly seen in elderly people. In an Argentinean study, 90 percent of the patients showed either favorable or very favorable response to ginseng therapy. These results are due to a measured increase in the blood flow in the cerebral and carotid arteries, which are the main arteries supplying blood to the brain. Scientists hypothesize that the positive effect of ginseng on the blood supply to the brain is due to its effect on the hypothalamus and the pituitary. Chemicals in these glands play a significant role in controlling many aspects of brain function.[6]

Dr. Petkov, Director of the Institute of Physiology of the Bulgarian Academy of Sciences, has been exploring the effects of ginseng on brain function, memory, and learning in laboratory animals. He states, "Ginseng stimulates the adrenal cortex, improves the ability to remember, accelerates learning, and even regulates the brain activity, placing it at a higher level."[7] The results of his studies show that ginseng treatment improved short-term memory, memory consolidation, and long-term memory.[8]

Another Russian study supported the work of Dr. Petkov, showing that extracts from Siberian ginseng exerted a positive influence on memory in mice.[9]

A German study investigated the effect of ginseng on the elderly. The researchers used Kraepelin's performance test to measure ginseng's ability to affect the quality and consistency of mental performance and concentration. This test is well known for its ability to provide very reliable information on age-specific brain functioning. The test provides exact measures of the subject's working behavior and reveals impairments of concentration and intellectual function. This study reported that ginseng significantly improved mental alertness, powers of concentration, ability to grasp abstract concepts, and general mental performance.[10]

There are hundreds of other studies demonstrating ginseng's ability to help the body recover from stress, to help problems with blood pressure, insomnia, menopause, cardiovascular disorders, cancer, and the immune system. Since we are focusing primarily on the enhancement of our mental functions, I will not detail them. I would, however, like to tell you a little about this remarkable plant, its origins, how it works and how to get it.

Origins

In Chinese, the word ginseng (jenshen) is written with the ideograms *jen* (gin), meaning man, and *seng*, meaning essence. The shape of the ginseng root often resembles the human form. The ancients believed that the spirit of God dwelled in these man-like roots, thus giving rise to such names as "Root of External Life," "Root of Life Plant," "Man's Health," and "Man's Root."

Ginseng is a short perennial herb. The upper part of this plant regenerates each year and reaches a height from seven to twenty-one inches. Each year's growth of leaves makes a scar on the plant stem that enables growers to determine the age of the plant. The ginseng root is creamy white or yellow and is harvested in the autumn after four to six years of growth. It is the root that contains the therapeutic properties.

Varieties of Ginseng

In A.D. 200, a Chinese emperor declared ginseng a "panacea." This gave rise to its botanical name *Panax ginseng*, which

Different Parts of the Ginseng Plant

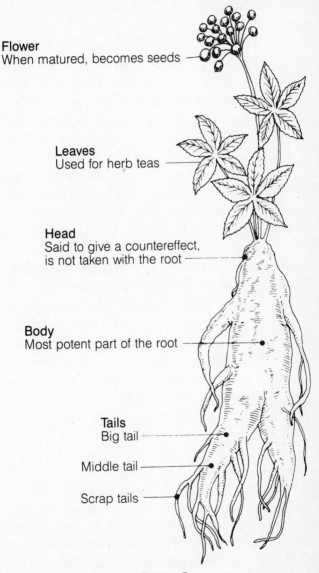

Flower
When matured, becomes seeds

Leaves
Used for herb teas

Head
Said to give a countereffect,
is not taken with the root

Body
Most potent part of the root

Tails
Big tail

Middle tail

Scrap tails

FIGURE 7.

actually originates from the Greek word meaning "cure-all" or "all-healing." *Panax ginseng* has become almost extinct in the wild but is cultivated widely in China, Japan, the U.S.S.R., and South Korea.

The North American variety of ginseng, *Panax quinquefolium*, grows wild in some areas in the Appalachians, northern United States, and sparsely, in Canada. Much to the dismay of wildcrafters, conservationists are exerting tight controls on this wild ginseng. Ginseng is also grown commercially in North America, primarily in Wisconsin. One county in Wisconsin expects to realize $25 million from a crop this year.

Siberian ginseng, or *Eleutherococcus senticosus*, is native to Russia and is actually a botanical cousin to *Panax ginseng*. It still can be found wild in Siberia and Japan and is grown commercially in the U.S.S.R., China, Korea, and Japan. Soviet researchers have devoted most of their attention to this variety. It is also the variety you will find in brain formulas and herbal preparations designed to stimulate mental functions.

The experts do not agree on which variety has the greatest potency and value. Some say *Panax ginseng* is the only "authentic" form of ginseng.[11] Others say the North American variety has been shown to have a greater concentration of saponins, the active ingredient.[12] Still others say that, because of the slight difference in the active ingredients, Siberian ginseng is the "prize of all ginseng breeds" and is the most effective and reliable adaptogen available.[13,14]

To further complicate matters, within each variety there are several levels of quality. For example, *Panax ginseng* roots are classified as heaven grade (first class), earth grade (second class) and man grade (third class). Heaven grade averages about $50 per ounce. Ginseng harvested from the wild remains the most desired and commands the greatest price. It sells anywhere from $3,000 to $10,000 per ounce and seldom leaves the country of its origin.

Growing Ginseng

The variations in the quality are directly related to soil conditions, the length of growing time, the extraction process, and the weather. It takes from four to six years for the ginseng root to reach full maturity. The younger roots have not concentrated enough of the active ingredients for therapeutic use. Six years is a significant amount of time to tie up agricultural land on one crop and it is sometimes a temptation to "force age" the root, thus reducing its potency.

Another fascinating aspect of this herb is its incredible appetite. The land is so depleted of its nutrients by a single crop of ginseng that another crop cannot be grown for ten to forty years. After a crop is harvested in Wisconsin, growers retire the land permanently and it is utilized for grazing or some other purpose not requiring high soil nutrition. One can begin to understand why ginseng is such a powerful herb and why it is expensive.

Processing Ginseng

There are several methods of processing the root: drying and steaming, boiling, and alcohol extraction. The creamy white to slightly yellow ginseng roots are usually cured by sun drying. Should you come into contact with a red variety of ginseng, it is simply regular white ginseng with its bark intact that has been boiled with other herbs for several hours and then cured in an oven or over a low fire.

The two curing procedures create a product with different smell, taste, color, and texture, but tests show that their biological activities are virtually the same. A common method of processing by the Koreans involves stripping the bark. This is unfortunate because the bark contains the highest content of the active ingredients. White ginseng may or may not have the bark stripped. Red ginseng always has the bark intact.

Active Ingredients

Scientific research has discovered that the medicinal or therapeutic properties of ginseng are due to a group of six chemicals called glycosides, also known as saponins or ginsenosides. As noted earlier, there is a tremendous variation in the levels of saponin content of ginseng roots and products containing ginseng. There are also variations of the active ingredients in the different types of ginseng. Standardized ginseng extracts that help solve this problem are now being produced.

Ginseng contains vitamins A, E, B-1 (thiamine), B-2 (riboflavin), B-3 (niacin) and B-12, folic acid, biotin, and ascorbic acid. It also contains the minerals iron, calcium, phosphorous, copper, magnesium, potassium, sulfur, manganese, germanium, cobalt, and sodium.

Scientists have gained a good understanding of the effects of these active ingredients that have the ability to inactivate free radicals and prevent biological damage.[15] They reduce the activation of the adrenal cortex, inhibiting the body's response to the alarm stage of stress.[16] The active ingredients increase the activity of the lymphocytes, which enhance the immune system.[17] The ingredients in ginseng also influence the metabolism of important neurotransmitters such as serotonin and acetylcholine that are important in mental functioning.[18]

In summary, the activities of the brain and the body require the expenditure of energy. It is the regulation of energy that underlies the biological action of the active ingredients of ginseng.[19]

How to Buy and Use Ginseng

The different kinds and qualities of ginseng can truly be overwhelming when you are trying to select the right product for yourself. I visited a comprehensive health food store to research what was currently available on the market. I learned from the very knowledgeable proprietor that the effects of the various types of products are as broad as the number of people using them. Choosing the best product ultimately becomes a matter of experimentation and learning your own biochemical needs.

Ginseng comes in the following forms:

1. Extracts
2. Pastes and granular teas
3. Pills, capsules, and tablets
4. Powders
5. Dried roots
6. Wines, liquors, gums, baked goods, etc.

Extracts and granular extract teas are the most easily absorbed, yet can be bitter in taste. Peppermint or honey can help make them palatable. Capsules are convenient, but one should take them with warm water to soften the cellulose that covers the ginseng powder. It will be helpful for those who chew the root to know that it is best not to chew off pieces of the root and swallow. Our digestive systems are incapable of breaking down the hard wood-like cellulose. Allowing the root to remain in the mouth for extended periods of time is the most effective way of gaining maximum absorption of the active ingredients. For maximum absorption, ginseng is best taken on an empty stomach.[20]

How do you know you are getting a potent product? This is an important issue to consider when buying ginseng. Good-grade ginseng is expensive. As a general rule, this is a product for which price determines quality. Top-quality ginseng begins in the $40 per ounce range. Midrange runs between $15 to $40. Your local health food store proprietor may be helpful in recommending products of known quality.

Dosage

Five hundred milligrams daily in divided doses has been reported to be therapeutically effective. The American Medical

Association recommends two to three grams per day for maximum therapeutic value. Greater quantities should be taken only under the care of a competent health professional.[21]

Contraindications

Individuals with high blood pressure should be cautious about using large quantities of ginseng. This is the only contraindication mentioned in the literature.

Final Comments

The primary value of ginseng appears to reside in its ability to function as an adaptogen. It is widely known for its ability to counteract many types of stress, both physical and mental. Ginseng's overall ability to modulate stress and other physical symptoms affecting mental performance makes it a valuable substance for promoting and sustaining clear thinking, sharp memory, and mental energy.

III

ANTIAGING

19

Introduction to Antiaging: Once a Dead Brain Cell, Always a Dead Brain Cell

In this section of *Mind Food and Smart Pills* we will focus on the nutrients and methods used for the maintenance of intelligence and mental capabilities. It is important not only to increase mental performance to optimal levels, but also to maintain this fine-tuned level of optimal performance throughout your entire lifetime.

I believe that future historians will document something that is happening now as one of the most significant milestones in the entire history of mankind. We are starting to understand the aging process, and we are learning how to control it. At this point in time we cannot begin to estimate how important this breakthrough will be to future generations.

When I talk about antiaging, I do not mean to infer that we will not age. Antiaging means slowing down and exercising control over the rate of aging. It also means slowing down the rate at which brain cells are damaged, which means delaying the onset of senility and/or preventing it from happening at all.

Some aspects of the aging process can even be reversed. The most dramatic example of this in terms of brain aging is the ability of the drug Lucidril (see Chapter 11) to dissolve and remove cellular garbage deposits in brain cells.

In addition to drug treatments, appropriate health-related changes in diet and life style can produce dramatic changes for most people. In a relatively short period of time you can actually "re-set" your biological age to more youthful levels.

Biological Aging Measurements

Measuring biological aging is a relatively new science. Several tests have been developed to measure different aspects of the aging process. The first time you take these tests you will get a comparison of your biological age with your chronological age. Then, when you take the test in the future, you can actually track your own rate of aging.

Some of the tests to determine biological age measure:

1. The functional capacity of the cardiovascular system
2. The immune system
3. Blood chemistries
4. The pulmonary system (lungs)
5. Vision and hearing

Some of the neuropsychological tests measure finger dexterity, hand steadiness, concentration, short-term memory, and reaction time, to name just a few. Measurements of body size and flexibility are recorded. These results are then put into a complex equation that produces the composite biological age of the individual being tested.[1]

The following example shows how dramatically the aging process can be reversed. This is a true story of a man I will refer to as Dr. J. Dr. J. was a thirty-nine-year-old professor on the faculty at the University of Arizona. His life style habits were poor and so was his health. He was overweight, he smoked cigarettes, he consumed alcohol regularly, and his diet was high in fast foods, sweets, coffee, and soft drinks. He began to feel so bad that it scared him. This prompted him to call a faculty friend and ask for some advice. The friend he called was involved with the testing and measuring of biological ages.

Dr. J. was put through the battery of biological tests and measurements. The results showed that thirty-nine-year-old Dr. J. had a biological age of sixty-one. This really scared him. He was told that if he didn't make some changes, he was a prime candidate for an early heart attack and possibly even death. Fortunately for Dr. J., his friend gave him some good advice on the types of changes he needed to make.

Dr. J. switched to a vegetarian diet and stopped his smoking and drinking. He also began to jog and eventually became a marathon runner. He dropped a tremendous amount of weight and became somewhat of a fanatic about health and exercise.

Three years later Dr. J. again went through biological age testing procedures. This time, at age forty-two, his biological age equaled that of a seventeen-year-old![2]

From: chronological age 39,   biological age 61

To: chronological age 42,   biological age 17

Granted, most people may not be interested in making this level of commitment to turning their lives around. However, I think it is an outstanding example of the degree to which we can reverse our biological age. And smaller changes in life style will still produce large changes in biological age.

How the Brain Ages

There are a number of ways that brain functions can deteriorate. A poor diet can result in damaged cellular structure in the neurons that in turn affects cell function and the rate of nerve transmissions. A suboptimal supply of blood and oxygen increases free radical damage to brain cells. Low levels of neurotransmitters affect memory. The accumulation of toxic metals such as lead, cadmium, and mercury can adversely affect memory, learning, and reasoning, leading to lower I.Q. scores. These problems, along with the other diseases of aging, can be prevented. The prevention of these problems is not a medical problem, it is an educational problem.

Health Education

I would like to make the need for better health education programs an issue of national concern. I propose that much more of our health care and medical research dollars be diverted to health education. Why chase after expensive cures when the problems can be prevented? The cure lies in prevention and prevention comes through education.

People make choices and changes when they understand the reason for doing so. Advice alone often misses the mark. "Take vitamin C twice daily," "don't eat margarine," "take extra selenium" are the types of things you may frequently hear. If you don't understand how important these suggestions are, or why they are important, chances are you will not follow the advice. People usually don't make changes unless they have a reason to do so. It is education about issues of health that provides us with understanding.

When you know about the toxic fats in margarine, you treat it like a poison. When you learn how selenium, vitamin C, and the other antioxidant nutrients protect you and slow down your rate of aging, you are likely to be inspired to make sure these nutrients are in your diet. When you know the difference and if you care about your life, it is not difficult to make choices in favor of health.

Building a New Body

Resetting your biological age to more youthful levels and reversing the aging process takes time. Over time, you are actually building a new body. Our society is programmed to want instant change. We tend to believe that when we feel bad all we have to do is go to the doctor, take a magic pill, and make the problem go away. People are always looking for a quick fix, the magic bullet.

Nutritional and biological therapies require time, commitment, and patience. You will be changing the functional capacity of enzyme systems. You will be changing biological processes. The body is gradually and continually turning over old cells and building new ones. When you start giving your body quality nutrition and exercise, the rebuilding and regeneration will take place naturally and gradually. Give the process from three to six months. You will look better on the outside, you will feel better on the inside. You will also have more energy and more enthusiasm for life. You are in the process of becoming a new person.

Recall how successfully Dr. J. reversed his biological aging process. Nevertheless, this example should not give us license to abuse ourselves. It is much easier to maintain the status of our health than it is to repair it. We do know that, with strong commitment, we can regenerate and repair most of the cells in our bodies. However, the same is not true of the human brain. Brain cells cannot be regenerated. Once a dead brain cell, always a dead brain cell.

The time to make a commitment to health is now. What you do today determines the body and mind you live with tomorrow.

It is my hope that the information in *Mind Food and Smart Pills* will provide a dimension of health education that is missing for many people. I wish to ignite a spark of excitement that inspires action. When I realized fully how total my responsibility is for my own health, intelligence, learning, and aging, it changed my life forever. Taking charge of your own life empowers you, it builds self-confidence and self-esteem. I am delighted to be able to share this information with you.

20

Optimal Nutrition and Intelligence

There is a growing body of research demonstrating that both diet and nutritional supplements have the ability to affect your intelligence and mental functions. Research also shows that a large percentage of our population, although not starving, is undernourished. The adequacy of the Standard American Diet (SAD) and the Recommended Daily Allowances (RDAs) is being challenged. Are they sufficient to maintain and optimize our intelligence and mental functioning?

Nutritional Supplements and I.Q.

In January 1988, *The Lancet* published a landmark study that showed a positive relationship between supplementation and I.Q. in British schoolchildren. This study is titled "Effect of Vitamin and Mineral Supplements on Intelligence of a Sample of School Children."

In this study, ninety British schoolchildren aged twelve and thirteen kept a diet diary for three days. It was found that some vitamins and numerous minerals were below RDA levels in the diet of many of these children.

For eight months, thirty of the students were given a multivitamin/mineral supplement, thirty were given a placebo, and the remaining thirty did not take any tablets. This study was designed to examine the possibility that deficiency of vitamins and minerals in the diet was preventing optimum psychological function.

At the end of the study, it was found that there was no difference in the three groups in verbal intelligence scores. However, the students who took the vitamin/mineral supplements registered significant increases in nonverbal intelligence scores. The placebo group and those who took no supplements registered no significant change.[1]

Having observed the diets of many teenage schoolchildren in the United States, I think the results from this British study should be a warning to us. The conclusion we can extrapolate from the results of this study is that dietary deficiencies hinder mental functioning in many schoolchildren, and that adequate nutritional supplementation can actually increase the intelligence of a nutritionally deficient child.

Nutrition and Academic Performance

The second study that I want to report here is vast in its scope, with equally staggering implications. The title of this study is "The Impact of a Low Food Additive and Sucrose Diet on Academic Performance in 803 New York City Public Schools."

From 1979 through 1983, the New York City Public School system instituted dietary revisions that produced remarkable positive effects on the academic achievement of the city's eight hundred thousand students.

The study reduced the amount of sugar, artificial food colors, artificial food flavors and preservatives in the meals served throughout the city schools. The changes were instituted gradually over the four-year period. Each year that a dietary improvement was made, significant improvement in citywide academic achievement was documented by comparing each school's standardized test scores with national averages. During year three of the study, no dietary changes were made and no academic improvement was made.

Before the dietary revisions, only about 1 percent variation occurred from year to year in the overall test scores for the city's 803 schools. Over the four years of the study with dietary improvements, the New York City schools raised their mean national academic scores 15.7 percent, with the gains only occurring during the first, second, and fourth years, coinciding with the years the dietary revisions were made.

Another interesting and important aspect of this study is that before the diet revisions were made, a negative association existed between the percentage of students eating school food and the overall academic test scores for that school. In other words, in schools where a higher percentage of the students ate school meals, the school's overall test scores were lower.

After the implementation of the dietary revisions, this situation reversed so that in the schools where a higher percentage of the students were eating healthy meals, the school's overall test scores were higher.

The results of a study of this magnitude make a strong statement about the relationship between nutrition and mental performance. This study indicates that the diet of our children may be contributing to a decrease in academic performance. Conversely, when improved diets are provided, students can make significant improvements in academic achievement.[2]

Optimal Nutrition

How do we know if we are receiving optimal nutrition? The two previous studies indicate that there is a significant relationship between diet, nutrition, and mental performance. What can we do to ensure that we are giving our minds and bodies the raw material they need for maximum performance?

Although most people are aware that there is an important connection between nutrition and health, but they are confused by the constant stream of conflicting information that bombards us in the press, in magazines, and on television.

For example, experts told us that we need more fiber to fight certain kinds of cancer. Then the FDA prevented cereal manufacturers from stating that fiber was useful in preventing these cancers. Other experts contended that the case for fiber is overstated. Now there are new findings that there are different types of fiber and not all fibers are equal.

The problem is that we get conflicting, technical, constantly changing recommendations from a host of experts. One day the government gives us Minimum Daily Requirements (MDRs). The next day we are told to forget that and concentrate on Recommended Daily Allowances (RDAs). We are told that we can get all we need from our diet and then told that we need supplements because our diet is inadequate. On top of it all we are told that needs vary from person to person and that the guidelines do not apply to everyone. It is no surprise that we are confused.

This chapter will give you a way of sorting through the competing claims and recommendations by explaining what the technical terms mean and by showing you how to make choices that can work for you.

The Minimum Daily Requirement

Let's begin our discussion by looking at the approved nutritional standards. The first set of guidelines, the Minimum Daily Requirements (MDRs), were issued by the U.S. Government as part of the post–World War II public health campaign. These standards set the minimal amounts necessary to prevent outright nutritional deficiency diseases. Examples are scurvy from lack of vitamin C, beriberi from lack of B-1, pellagra from niacin deficiency, rickets from vitamin D deficiency.

Most doctors and health professionals agree that vitamin deficiency diseases have ceased to be major health problems. They are no longer encountered in the major health surveys conducted in the United States. In fact, they are so rare in this country that they reside somewhere between medical curiosity and historical fact.

There is a level of nutrition implied in the MDR-deficiency. When we are not getting enough of one or more nutrients we are functioning at the deficient level. Severe deficiency is rarely met in this country, but moderate and undetected deficiencies are more common than suspected. The problem is that severe deficiencies are very dramatic. Your teeth fall out, your bones become soft, you break out in ulcers. Slight deficiencies may make you moody, sluggish, or more susceptible to colds, and their underlying nutritional deficiencies can go undetected.

The Recommended Daily Allowances

Today the MDR has been replaced by the Recommended Daily Allowances (RDAs). These guidelines were developed by the Food and Nutrition Board of the National Academy of Sciences/National Research Council (NAS/NRC). The RDA guidelines represent the "recommendations for the average daily amounts of nutrients that population groups should consume over a period of time." Notice the wording here. The RDAs do not represent individual requirements. They are statistical averages for the population at large. This means that they do not apply to each individual. Some people will need more and some will need less.

The RDAs are set somewhat higher than the MDRs. In this way the government standards virtually ensure that people meeting the RDAs in their diets will not get vitamin deficiency diseases. But even the experts disagree on the RDAs. Two years ago the National Research Council announced that it would be unable to issue the scheduled tenth edition of the RDA. The authors and researchers disagreed with each other so strongly that the scheduled revision of the RDAs has been suspended indefinitely!

Much of this controversy centers around an important philosophical question that inspires emotionally charged debates. The issue is the difference between adequate and optimal levels of nutrition.

The Optimal Daily Requirement

The term "Optimal Daily Requirement" (ODR) has been coined here to describe a level of nutrition that meets the need for the optimal health of an individual instead of merely avoiding deficiency diseases. So far the guidelines issued by the government are designed to prevent disease. But what about meeting our needs for optimal health?

We can get a deeper understanding of this question by taking a close look at the health of this nation. As a nation, we have the highest level of chronic degenerative diseases such as cardiovascular problems, arthritis, and cancer. Physical aging and mental deterioration are America's primary health problems. Heart disease kills 52 percent of the people in the country. One in every three develops cancer. The World Health Organization estimates that about 80 percent of the deaths in the United States result from chronic degenerative diseases.

Although it is a controversial position, many health experts agree that degenerative diseases have underlying nutritional deficiencies associated with them. There is substantial research that indicates that good nutrition and sound health practices can prevent many chronic degenerative diseases.

The level of nutrition that prevents chronic degenerative disease and promotes optimal health is called the Optimal Daily Requirement. It is my sincere belief that heart disease, cancer, arthritis, and senility can be prevented through optimal nutrition and good sound health practices such as regular, moderate exercise. I believe the RDAs are out-of-date because they are set too low for the promotion of health. Much evidence indicates that adherence to the current RDA guidelines will ensure poor health later in life. Instead of emphasis on simply preventing scurvy and other deficiency diseases, we need to focus on what it takes to create optimal health and wellness. Let's eliminate chronic degenerative disease at its source.

Excess Levels of Nutrition

It is possible to get too much of a good thing. We need protein and fat in our diet, but the average American diet includes far too much of both. We need carbohydrates, especially the complex carbohydrates in potatoes and other starchy foods. But we Americans eat far too much sugar and other simple carbohydrates like corn syrup. This is nutrition at the excess level. It results in what is known as overconsumption and undernutrition, leading to too many calories with too little nutrient value.

We can get too much of other nutrients, such as vitamins A, E, and D. These are fat-soluble vitamins like vitamin C. However, these excesses are extremely rare, especially in comparison to the common excess levels of fat and sugar.

We have looked at five levels of nutrition:
1. The deficient level
2. The minimum daily requirement
3. The recommended daily requirement
4. The optimal daily requirement
5. The excess level

Each succeeding level represents an increase in the level of nutrition, but more isn't necessarily better. Now that we have defined the five levels of nutrition we are ready to look at the importance of choice in diet and health.

Choice in Nutrition

We do not have to be slaves to the guidelines issued by governmental agencies or even to the recommendations of individual experts. We have freedom of choice, and nutrition is one of the most important areas in which we can exercise choices.

There are no final answers in the area of nutrition. There is no perfect expert or panel of experts that can tell us exactly what to do. We have to gather in the available information and make the best decision possible based on that information.

The first question each of us has to decide is the level of health that is satisfactory. One person may be willing to smoke, avoid all exercise, and eat plenty of fats. That is a prescription for an early death from heart disease or some other degenerative disease, but it is a choice that an individual in this country is free to make. Another person may not want to be bothered with learning about nutrition and health. In that case the government-issued RDAs are fine and no more effort is desired.

But since you are reading this book you probably want to live at a level of health that is above the bare minimum. You are interested in learning about the latest research and its meaning in your life. But you still have to make choices based on the information you get about a wide range of nutrients.

Essential Nutrients

What constitutes a healthy diet? What do we really need to be healthy and to stay healthy? Research has discovered that there are at least forty-five essential nutrients. "Essential" means that our bodies are incapable of manufacturing these nutrients, and we must get them from the foods we eat or from nutritional supplements.

For example, the body cannot manufacture the vitamins from other food sources. Sailors developed scurvy because a diet of crackers and dried beef does not contain any vitamin C. When it was discovered that citrus fruit prevented scurvy, the British navy started adding lime juice to the daily allowance of rum, hence the name "Limey" for British sailors.

But the question remains, "What constitutes a healthy diet?" As a simplified guideline to a balanced diet the concept of the four major food groups was developed. These are meat or fish, dairy, grains, and vegetables. Evidence about the sources of chronic diseases have led many nutritionists to recommend cutting down on salt and fat intake, which means less meat and dairy. Some say complex carbohydrates are important and others emphasize getting plenty of protein—although most evidence indicates that the American diet is excess in protein. Others advocate vegetarian diets. Since the experts cannot agree, you have to gather the evidence and make the choices that are right for you and the life you want to live.

You may decide to eliminate meat from your diet or you may decide you just cannot give up hamburgers. You can decide to increase the level of fiber in your diet or you can decide the best thing for you in the morning is coffee and a doughnut. It is important for you to make an *informed* decision, but the choice is yours.

Before reviewing some general recommendations about diet, there is one more issue to look at—individual variation in dietary needs.

Individual Nutritional Needs

Dr. Roger Williams, often referred to as the father of modern nutrition, addressed the issue of individual nutritional needs in his classic paper "Biochemical Individuality."[3] He postulated that although we all function on the same biological principles, we are all biologically unique. He pointed out that one person's need for any given nutrient may be ten to one hundred times greater than another person's. Individual variations in nutritional requirements can have serious consequences if the needs are not understood and met.

How many times have all the people around you had severe colds or flu and you were not touched? Or the opposite? Some people eat well, exercise, and still get sick. Why? The reasons and variables are endless and very individualistic. Most people have genetic traits that predispose them to illness or health.

Different levels of stress lead to different levels of nutritional need. Your nutritional needs are different from those of other people and they vary from day to day.

The point is that your own personal nutritional requirements cannot possibly be met by following the guidelines for the statistically average person. Your nutritional needs are different from those of everyone else and those needs vary from day to day. How can you find your individual nutritional needs?

The answer is that you have to experiment. The guidelines such as the RDA give you the beginning of an answer. But to find your individual optimal level of nutrition you have to vary the amount of different nutrients and discover what works for you. Increasing the level of B vitamins you take may improve your mood and enable you to deal with stress or it may have no noticeable effect. Less protein and fat may give you a lighter feeling or may leave you feeling empty and hungry. Substituting complex carbohydrates for sugar snacks may eliminate the low energy period that can result from the body's attempt to get the excess sugar out of the bloodstream.

To find the optimal level of nutrition for you as an individual, you have to gather information about nutrition and then experiment for yourself to discover what works for you.

Basic Guidelines

I feel that I would be shirking my responsibility in this discussion about diet if I did not give some basic guidelines that, in my opinion, can serve as the foundation of a healthy diet.

Raw fruits, vegetables, whole grains, beans, and seeds are the backbone of a healthy diet. Notice that I did not mention animal products. Research indicates that animal fats contribute to chronic degenerative disease. Although I do recommend a diet free from animal products, I also understand that it would require a dramatic change in lifestyle for most people to completely eliminate them from their diets. If you eat dairy products, keep them low-fat. If you eat meat, it is advisable to concentrate on fish. Other lean meats should be organically raised because of the antibiotics and hormones that are added to their feed.

This diet is high in fiber, complex carbohydrates, vitamins and minerals, while it is low in fat and avoids excess protein. But there remains an important question. Even if you focus on selecting fresh fruits, vegetables, and other natural and unprocessed foods, will you be able to get the level of nutrients you need for optimal health and wellness?

Factory Farming

There has been a major change in our food supply system and the food it delivers to us in the last fifty years. We have shifted from an agricultural food supply to an industrial food supply. It begins at the farming end and is referred to as factory farming. Genetic manipulation, fertilization, and pesticide use greatly alter the basic foods that are produced. Animals are given large doses of antibiotics and hormones to speed growth. Then they are artificially fattened on grain to increase their weight.

Foods are force ripened, picked early, frozen, and stored. They are then shipped to the giant food processing industries. The food is sweetened. Fat, preservatives, and other chemicals are added. The food may even be irradiated. Our food supply is controlled by giant corporations that control millions of farm acres and decide the fate of our food supply from beginning to end. The primary interest of these corporations is profit, and there is little interest in the nutritional content of the end product.

The food in your neighborhood grocery store may look fresh, but how nutritious is it? The chart below shows the tremendous range in the nutritional content in a number of fruits and vegetables. A tomato may look, feel, and taste good, but you

Variations in Mineral Content in Vegetables

	Total Ash or Mineral Matter	Percentage of Dry Weight			Millequivalents per 100 Grams Dry Weight			Trace Elements Parts per Million Dry Matter			
		Phosphorus	Calcium	Magnesium	Potassium	Sodium	Boron	Manganese	Iron	Copper	Cobalt
SNAP BEANS											
Highest	10.45	0.36	40.5	60.0	99.7	8.6	73	60	227	69	0.26
Lowest	4.04	0.22	15.5	14.8	29.1	0.0	10	2	10	3	0.00
CABBAGE											
Highest	10.38	0.38	60.0	43.6	148.3	20.4	42	13	94	48	0.15
Lowest	6.12	0.18	17.5	15.6	53.7	0.8	7	2	20	0.4	0.00
LETTUCE											
Highest	24.48	0.43	71.0	49.3	176.5	12.2	37	169	516	60	0.19
Lowest	7.01	0.22	6.0	13.1	53.7	0.0	6	1	9	3	0.00
TOMATOES											
Highest	14.20	0.35	23.0	59.2	148.3	6.5	36	68	1938	53	0.63
Lowest	6.07	0.16	4.5	4.5	58.8	0.0	5	1	1	0	0.00
SPINACH											
Highest	28.56	0.52	96.0	203.9	257.0	69.5	88	117	1584	32	0.25
Lowest	12.38	0.27	47.5	46.9	84.6	0.8	12	1	19	0.5	0.20

(Firman E. Bear report. Rutgers U.)

FIGURE 8.

are playing Russian roulette with your long-term health unless you become conscious of the real food value in it. There are many studies showing that most Americans are not even meeting the RDA level of nutrition.

The other major issue is the total level of environmental stress that most people are exposed to in our society. Mental and emotional stress burns up essential nutrients like vitamin C and the B vitamins at a higher rate. Environmental stress from air pollution, toxins in food and water, and noise pollution make demands on our bodies. These pressures act as "vitamin robbers" and leave us open to emotional collapse and disease. The greater the stress, the higher the level of nutrition needed to withstand and counteract the many sources of stress in modern society.

Artificially altered food supply and the stress in our lives combine to rob people of the nutrients they need. Is it possible to meet these needs with improved selection of foods or do we need supplements?

Nutritional Supplements

I have been asked why we cannot get all the nutrients we need from a balanced diet if our ancestors lived off the land and needed no supplements. They sometimes add that their doctors have told them that vitamins only create expensive urine. An interesting study, "Paleolithic Nutrition," shows that the diet of our ancestors was superior to the current food supply in some very important ways. First of all, the vitamin intake of prehistoric humans substantially exceeded ours. They also consumed less fat and ate a lower percentage of saturated fats. The study concluded that the diet of our remote ancestors could serve as a reference standard for modern human nutrition and a model for defense against many of today's chronic degenerative diseases.[4]

Because of the evidence that our food supply is lacking in

some essential nutrients and because of the added demands of stressful living, I am a strong advocate of nutritional supplementation. I believe everyone should take a high-potency multivitamin/mineral supplement daily. I am not talking about supermarket one-a-day vitamins that are based on the outmoded RDA guidelines. High-potency formulations contain more vitamins and minerals than can fit into our tablet or capsule. The recommended daily dosage in the higher-potency nutritional supplements will usually be two or more tablets or capsules per day.

How much of each nutrient should you take? That is a difficult question because we have never been able to test what nutrient levels are necessary for optimal health.

Biochemical individuality plays a critical role in deciding how much to take. I may only require 3000 milligrams of vitamin C per day, but my wife may need 5000 due to the stresses of her work. Also, due to the physiological differences, a woman may need a higher level of calcium or iron than the average man.

The pursuit of optimal health is a never-ending detective story in which you find out about your biochemical uniqueness and then learn how to satisfy your own nutritional needs. Our bodies are made from a combination of food, air, and water. If something is wrong with your health, look first to these areas for the answer.

In the following chapters, I hope to give you enough information on how to strengthen the immune system and use antiaging nutrients so that you can begin your own personal quest for optimal health and wellness.

21

Vitamin C/Ascorbic Acid: The Champion Free Radical Scavenger

This is the first of several nutrients that may help to retard or prevent brain aging. The aging process does not have to lead to senility and loss of memory. By preventing the damage that free radicals can cause and by protecting the integrity of the cell walls of the neurons, we can continue to enjoy the full use of our mental faculties as long as we live.

Vitamin C is a multipurpose ally and you should know it as intimately as you would a best friend. It should be a constant companion, and in turn, it will do wonders for you. From colds to cancer, vitamin C plays an active role in protection and prevention.

Close to a miracle substance, vitamin C:

1. Protects against and reduces the severity of colds and flu in some people.
2. Speeds wound healing.
3. Reduces the duration and frequency of herpes infections.
4. Is an excellent natural antihistamine.
5. Helps protect against cardiovascular disease.
6. Is a potent detoxifier and protects against environmental pollutants.
7. Reduces anxiety and promotes sleep.
8. Enhances mental alertness.

Vitamin C helps to build strong connective tissue (collagen). In fact, collagen can't be formed without vitamin C. Collagen is responsible for the strength of bones, teeth, skin, tendons, blood vessels, and other parts of the body. The gradual deterioration of collagen is directly related to the aging process.

Nature has given most animals the ability to manufacture all the vitamin C they need. However, through a quirk of evolutionary fate, humans lack the enzyme that enables us to synthesize vitamin C from glucose. This means that we have to get all of our vitamin C from our daily diet.

Vitamins occur in two forms, water-soluble and fat-soluble. Water-soluble vitamins are not stored in the body and are eliminated in the urine. Fat-soluble vitamins are stored in the body for longer periods of time. Since vitamin C is water-soluble, our bodies cannot store it; excesses are excreted in the urine. After taking vitamin C (either in your food or as a vitamin supplement), its biological effect only lasts about six hours. Thus, for high-level wellness and optimal antioxidant protection, humans need to replenish their bodies with supplies of this most essential antioxidant vitamin *several times a day*.

Effects

Vitamin C is one of the most important and effective antioxidant protectors in the human body. It is the body's principal circulating antioxidant. When we have adequate levels of vitamin C, it is carried by the blood throughout the body and "bathes" the cells with protection. When a free radical appears, a vitamin C molecule sacrifices one of its own electrons to neutralize the invader. Each time this occurs, vitamin C is destroyed and the body's supply of vitamin C is depleted, but vulnerable cells in the body are saved. This battle between harmful free radicals and vitamin C takes place hundreds of thousands (maybe millions) of times each second, depending on your rate of metabolism and the amount of vitamin C available in your body.[1]

The Vitamin C Pump

The brain and spinal cord (collectively called the central nervous system) are the most important parts of the body. Nature provides a special protective mechanism to protect these areas. This mechanism is known as *the vitamin C pump*.

The central nervous system contains the highest concentration of fat of any organ in the body. The types of fats that make up the cells in the CNS are more highly unsaturated than fats in other areas of the body. This makes the cells of the central nervous system much more vulnerable to oxidation and free radical damage.

The vitamin C pump has two parts. The first part extracts vitamin C from the circulating blood and increases its concentration by a factor of ten in the cerebrospinal fluid. The second part extracts vitamin C from the cerebrospinal fluid and concentrates it by another factor of ten around the nerve cells of the brain and spinal cord. Nature protects the cells of the brain and spinal cord by "bathing" them in vitamin C that is one hundred times more concentrated than in normal body fluids.[2]

Vitamin C and Intelligence

A study done on patients in a British hospital dramatically demonstrated the relationship of vitamins to mental function. The study found many cases where geriatric patients were suffering from mental confusion due to vitamin C deficiency. The simple addition of vitamin C supplements caused remarkable improvements. In another controlled study, students with higher vitamin C levels scored an average of five points higher on IQ tests than those with lower vitamin C levels. When the group with low vitamin C levels was given vitamin C supplements for six months, their IQ scores increased by 3.54 points.[3]

The Therapeutic Use of Vitamin C

Dr. William Cathcart has pioneered the use of extremely high doses of vitamin C to treat infections. He observed that about 80 percent of his patients normally could tolerate ten to fifteen grams of crystalline vitamin C orally in a twenty-four-hour period without developing diarrhea. However, the same patients when stressed by infection could greatly increase their vitamin C intake without producing diarrhea. Dr. Cathcart discovered that vitamin C was actually being used up fighting the infection, and that the sicker a person was, the greater the need for vitamin C. He also observed that his patients did not benefit from high-dose vitamin C therapy unless they ingested enough to bring them close to causing diarrhea (their bowel tolerance).

Dr. Cathcart calls this method of determining correct dosage levels "titrating to bowel tolerance." In the medical journal *Medical Hypotheses*, he explained,

> The maximum relief of symptoms which can be expected with oral doses of ascorbic acid is obtained at a point just short of the amount which produces diarrhea. This amount and the timing of the doses are usually sensed by the patient. The physician should not try to regulate exactly the amount and timing of these doses because the optimally effective dose will often change from dose to dose . . . the patient tries to titrate between that amount which begins to make him feel better and that amount which almost but not quite causes diarrhea.[4]

Occasionally, in a very severe infection, Dr. Cathcart will utilize the controlled intravenous administration of vitamin C. The following chart is a summary of the amounts of vitamin C Dr. Cathcart has found to be effective for various conditions.

I have recommended this therapy to many of my clients and friends and I have one note of advice to add to Dr. Cathcart's

Approximate Amounts of Vitamin C Required to Reach Bowel Tolerance for Various Conditions

Condition	Grams per 24 Hours	Number of Doses per 24 Hours
Normal	4 – 15	4 –
Mild cold	30 – 60	6 – 10
Severe cold	60 – 100	8 – 15
Influenza	100 – 150	8 – 20
Mononucleosis	150 – 200 +	12 – 25
Viral pneumonia	150 – 200 +	12 – 25
Hay fever, asthma	15 – 50	4 – 8
Environmental, food allergy	0.5 – 50	4 – 8
Burn, injury, surgery	25 – 150	6 – 20
Cancer	15 – 100	4 – 15
Rheumatoid arthritis	15 – 100	4 – 15
Bacterial infections	30 – 200 +	10 – 25
Infectious hepatitis	30 – 100	6 – 15
Candida infections	15 – 200 +	6 – 25
Anxiety, exercise, and other mild stresses	15 – 25	4 – 6

FIGURE 9.

regime. I find that people who follow this therapy throughout a day will improve quickly. Frequently, however, they wake up sick again the next day. What has happened is that the vitamin C is depleted fighting the infection during the night, and the virus is able to reestablish itself. Thus I recommend that people take a big dose just before going to bed at night. They should keep a jug of water and a supply of vitamin C on the night stand next to the bed. The alarm should be set to wake up twice during the night to take a large dose of vitamin C. The results will be far more effective.

Food Sources

When considering foods that contain vitamin C, bear in mind that the vitamin is volatile. Its concentration is highest when food is fresh, and it is depleted soon after harvest. Cooking also destroys much of the vitamin C content in foods.

Foods that are very high in vitamin C content are: broccoli, black currants, kale, parsley, and peppers. Foods that are high in vitamin C content are: brussels sprouts, cabbage, cauliflower, chives, collards, and mustard greens. Foods that are intermediate in vitamin C content are: artichokes, asparagus, beet greens, cantaloupe, lemons, limes, oranges, radishes, spinach, zucchini, strawberries, swiss chard, and ripe tomatoes.

In a good, healthy diet where attention is given to fresh, organic produce, I estimate an average vitamin C intake to be from 200 mg to 250 mg daily. The average American probably only gets about 50 mg. Nutritionally oriented health professionals recommend 1000 to 3000 mg per day. Clearly, supplementation is necessary for optimal health and protection.

Supplements

Vitamin C is available as regular tablets, time-release tablets, chewable tablets, and in powder form. The regular and time-release tablets are common and acceptable supplements. However, there is one note of caution. If vitamin C tablets are compressed too hard during manufacturing, they take longer to dissolve. A tablet may settle on the lining of the stomach while dissolving and cause a local inflammation or ulceration.

Chewing the vitamin C chewable tablets also warrants caution. Vitamin C is an acid (ascorbic acid). Over time, the ascorbic acid may begin to dissolve the protective enamel of the teeth.

There are several different forms of vitamin C available. The most common form of vitamin C is ascorbic acid, which is the acidic form of the vitamin. Calcium ascorbate and sodium ascorbate are other forms of vitamin C. The calcium and sodium salts are less acidic, which makes them more palatable for some people. (Sodium ascorbate should not be taken by those who have blood pressure problems or those who are on a low-salt diet).

Ascorbic acid and the calcium and sodium ascorbate salts are all easily ordered or purchased in bulk powder form. Buying vitamin C in bulk powder form is easier on both your stomach and your pocket book. The powdered forms are readily soluble and easily absorbed. It is also much more cost effective to buy vitamin C in bulk powder. For example, a kilogram (2.2 pounds) of ascorbic acid can be purchased from mail order sources for about $16.00. The equivalent amount of ascorbic acid purchased as regular vitamin C tablets would be about four to five times more expensive! In the powdered forms, one fourth of a teaspoon equals approximately 1000 mg or 1 gm of vitamin C.

NOTE: When exposed to air, ascorbic acid will oxidize to dehydroascorbate, which is toxic. Therefore when using vitamin C powder, it is important to mix it up fresh each time.

Ascorbyl Palmitate

Ascorbyl palmitate is a fat-soluble form of vitamin C. Because of its solubility in fats, it is more effective than water-soluble forms of vitamin C as an antioxidant in preventing lipid peroxidation. Ascorbyl palmitate is also more effective in transporting vitamin C into the fatty structures of the heart, brain, and central nervous system, protecting these organs from free radical damage. It is a powerful protector of fat-containing tissues and can be purchased in most health food stores.

Natural vs. Synthetic

Consumers are often confused by the controversy over the effectiveness of natural versus synthetic vitamins. There are two points to be made about the use of the word "natural" in this context. First, most synthetic vitamins are as effective as the natural forms (vitamin E is an exception). Synthetic vitamin C is cheaper and is essentially the same as the natural form.[5] Second, the term "natural" is frequently applied to vitamins as a marketing ploy rather than as a guide to the effective use of nutritional supplements. Frequently, a so-called "natural" product is mostly synthetic and contains only a small amount of the natural ingredient. For example, products labeled NATURAL VITAMIN C WITH ROSE HIPS are almost entirely synthetic vitamin C with a tiny pinch of rose hips powder added.

In nature, a group of compounds called bioflavonoids (sometimes called vitamin P) are produced with vitamin C. The bioflavonoids increase the effectiveness of vitamin C. Therefore, it is a good idea to take bioflavonoids along with vitamin C.

Dosage Range

The government RDA for vitamin C is 45 mg daily. However, according to many nutritionally oriented health professionals, a general range of vitamin C supplementation for adults is from 1 to 3 grams daily (1000 to 3000 mg/day), in divided doses.

Actually, we should not think in terms of a specific dosage of vitamin C as being "the correct dosage." Needs vary dramatically from person to person, and from day to day. Requirements will vary with age, levels of stress, and basic genetic differences.

Deficiency Symptoms

Bleeding gums and easy bruising are two classic signs of vitamin C deficiency. If you have these symptoms, take note of what your body is trying to tell you. Other conditions that can be associated with vitamin C deficiency are aching joints, fatigue, confusion, depression, and anemia. Some cases of infertility in men have been shown to be related to low vitamin C levels. Their sperm motility improved as their serum levels of vitamin C increased.

Vitamin C Robbers

We think in terms of nutrients for our bodies, but few of us stop to think about the antinutrients in our environment. There are a number of factors that rob vitamin C from us. Each cigarette smoked destroys approximately 25 mg of vitamin C; air pollution depletes vitamin C. The following types of drugs deplete vitamin C: antihistamines, aspirin, barbiturates, cortisone, and Indocin. Vitamin C is needed to make some of the body's stress hormones. Any kind of stress, physical, mental, or emotional will deplete vitamin C. Women taking birth control pills need higher levels of vitamin C. Also, exposure to heat, light, oxygen, and cooking will destroy vitamin C.

Side Effects

Gastritis, gas, and diarrhea seem to be the only unpleasant side effects from taking too much vitamin C. These problems are easily controlled by simply adjusting the dosage. Actually, the first sign of slight diarrhea (soft stools) is a desirable indicator. This is called your *bowel tolerance*, and it indicates that your body tissues are saturated with vitamin C.

Toxicity

One of the most remarkable qualities of vitamin C is its high level of safety over a very wide dosage range. It has been estimated that one would have to consume several pounds of vitamin C to reach a lethal dose. Reports claiming that large doses of vitamin C destroy vitamin B-12 have been found to be without scientific basis. Vitamin C has never been shown to destroy vitamin B-12 in the human body, only in a laboratory test tube. The claim that vitamin C will cause kidney stones is also unfounded. Levels of up to 10,000 mg a day in normal individuals showed no signs of kidney stone formation.

Rebound Effect

In a person taking higher amounts of vitamin C, many enzymes that utilize vitamin C are also produced in greater quantity. This allows the body to make greater use of the extra vitamin C that is available. If an individual taking regular large doses of vitamin C abruptly stops, a rebound effect can result. Blood ascorbate levels would drop, and the body's level of resistance would be lowered for one to two weeks. Therefore, if an individual who has been taking regular doses of vitamin C decides to revert to lower doses, it is advisable to decrease the intake gradually over a one- to two-week period.

Pregnant women who are taking larger doses of vitamin C should be aware of this rebound effect. The newborn baby could develop this rebound effect unless it is given vitamin C supplementation. Although greater quantities of nutrients are necessary during pregnancy, megadoses should never be taken without the close supervision of a physician.

Final Comments

Dr. Linus Pauling is one of America's most acclaimed scientists and the only two-time winner of the Nobel Prize. His research has convinced him that, in society as a whole, a 10 percent improvement in both physical and mental health can result from increased intake of vitamin C. Obviously, additional vitamin C will not make the same improvement in every individual. But the evidence for improvement in health and intelligence as a result of vitamin C supplementation is growing.

Although vitamin C is effective when taken therapeutically, its real benefit comes from being used on a daily basis. When used in this manner, it provides general protection against disease, and this is the way it should be utilized.

22

Selenium: The Miracle Element

Selenium is one of the most important nutritional discoveries of the twentieth century. It is a nutrient that no individual can afford to overlook. Every one of the 60,000,000,000,000 (sixty trillion) cells in your body needs a small amount of selenium in order to be protected and function properly. Selenium is becoming a nutritional "superstar." It is critical to good health.

Let us take a look at why selenium is so important. It is crucial to the functioning of one of the most important antioxidant enzyme systems in your body. It is the strongest anticancer nutrient known. It protects against heart and circulatory diseases. It is a powerful stimulant to the immune system. It aids in the removal of toxic metals and possesses strong anti-inflammatory properties.

Selenium and Toxic Metals

Toxic metals affect the brain and nervous system before they affect the other organs of the body, just as many nutritional deficiencies do. Selenium is one of the most powerful detoxifiers of poisonous heavy metals.

The toxic metals we most frequently are exposed to are mercury, lead, arsenic, and cadmium. These metals are absorbed into our systems through the food we eat, the air we breathe, and the water we drink. Our modern industrial society is environmentally much more toxic than in any other time in history. For example, studies show that we have accumulated approximately one thousand times more lead in our bodies than people living sixteen hundred years ago.[1]

Just how dangerous are these toxic heavy metals? A minuscule amount of any one of these substances can create serious distortions in brain chemistry. For example, small amounts of lead cause hyperactivity, learning disorders, and mental retardation. It is well known that children with higher lead accumulation have lower IQ scores. Removing lead has been shown to increase IQ scores.[2]

Mercury has a particular affinity for brain tissue. It causes a wide variety of psychological complaints, depression, irritability, and a failure of concentration. Some early symptoms are fatigue, headache, and forgetfulness. Some of the later symptoms are speech disorders, hearing difficulties, and loss of memory.

The brain is damaged by these toxic metals that displace some of the important minerals like iron, zinc, and copper in the brain's normal chemical reactions. Selenium binds to the toxic metals and removes them from the body.

Selenium and the Immune System

Selenium has been shown to boost significantly the immune system when it is given in amounts greater than ordinary nutritional requirements.[3] The body's antibody defenses have been shown to increase up to thirtyfold following the administration of a combination of selenium and vitamin E. Two other indexes of the immune system, phagocyte activity and lymphocyte activity, both improve with increased selenium and are depressed with selenium deficiency. This evidence indicates that selenium is very important to an optimally functioning immune system and one's ability to resist disease.

Selenium and Heart Disease

Selenium is also protective against heart disease and other cardiovascular problems. In mainland China, selenium has successfully eradicated a disease of national concern. Keshan's disease was killing the children of China. The disease is characterized by enlarged hearts and high death rates. It was discovered that the disease was occurring primarily in those areas where the selenium levels in the soil are particularly low. Knowledge of the importance of selenium supplementation has virtually eliminated the disease.[4]

Numerous population studies have shown that many forms of heart disease increase as the level of selenium decreases. There is an area in the United States called the "stroke belt" that encompasses part of the state of Georgia and the Carolinas. The soil in this area has been found to be very low in selenium content. The people living in this area have the highest rate of strokes in the United States as well as a very high incidence of cardiovascular disease.

Selenium and Cancer

Selenium has the potential to become a primary nutrient in the battle against cancer. Volumes of animal studies confirm selenium's anticancer properties, while population studies continue to affirm its protective role against various types of cancer in humans. There are several excellent reviews for readers desiring more in-depth information on selenium's anticancer capabilities.

I would like to refer to one aspect of selenium and cancer because it is research with which I was personally involved. I worked under Dr. Gerhard Schrauzer at the University of California at San Diego (UCSD) studying selenium's role in breast cancer.

We used a strain of female mice that were developed specifically for laboratory research. These mice had been infected with a cancer virus that was passed from the mother to the pups through the mother's milk. From 95 to 100 percent of the mice spontaneously developed cancer in their normal lifetimes. The tumor model that we used is particularly relevant to human breast cancer because some of the biochemical mechanisms are essentially the same.

When we added supplemental selenium to the diets of the mice, there was a tremendous reduction in the development of mammary tumors. Selenium supplementation reduced the rate of cancer incidence eightfold! Dr. Schrauzer has developed a worldwide reputation for his work on selenium and cancer. He has stated publicly that, if every woman in the United States would take 250 to 350 micrograms of selenium daily as a supplement, we would see a dramatic reduction in breast cancer in a very short time.[5]

Effects

Selenium is an essential trace element. It functions as part of the body's defense system because of its relationship to an enzyme named glutathione peroxidase. Glutathione peroxidase, as discussed in chapter 4, is a powerful antioxidant enzyme that protects cell membranes and tissues against free radical destruction. Each molecule of this important antioxidant enzyme contains four atoms of selenium. Thus, suboptimal selenium levels decreases the body's ability to manufacture glutathione peroxidase. This puts the whole immune system at risk and decreases resistance to disease.

Selenium also acts as an antioxidant on its own. Selenium magnifies the effectiveness of vitamin E. In turn, researchers have discovered, particularly in their work with cancer, that selenium is far more effective when used in conjunction with vitamin E.[6]

Selenium Deficiency

There are several reasons why we do not get adequate levels of selenium in our diets. A major reason is that humans and animals need selenium for healthy growth but plants do not. This means that plants can be perfectly healthy without selenium. Since there are no signs of selenium deficiency in plants, farmers do not add it to the soil, and the soil depletion of selenium continues to get worse.

Modern fertilization practices and acid rains reduce a plant's ability to incorporate selenium, even in the areas where the soil contains enough of this vital element.

The soil in many parts of the United States (and many parts of the world) is deficient in selenium. Food grown in these regions is low in selenium.

Food Sources

Food sources containing the highest amounts of selenium are whole-grain products, wheat germ, whole-grain breads and cereals, bran, and barley. Some types of fish also contain significant amounts of selenium, notably shellfish, tuna, and herring. Organ meats such as liver and kidney are also prime sources. There are traces of selenium in eggs, leafy green vegetables, asparagus, peanuts, brewer's yeast, and tomatoes. Keep in mind that the levels of selenium in these sources can vary due to regional differences to selenium in the soil.

Supplements

Selenium supplements are available in most health food stores and vitamin centers at reasonable prices. They come in strengths ranging from 25 mcg to 200 mcg per tablet.

Selenium supplements are available in two different forms, organic and inorganic. *The form of supplemental selenium you take is important*. Organically-bound selenium is produced commercially by growing yeast cells in a selenium-rich nutrient medium. The selenium is biologically incorporated into the yeast as it grows. Nutritional supplements made from the high selenium yeast are better absorbed and are ten to twenty times

Regional Selenium Content in Soil Classification

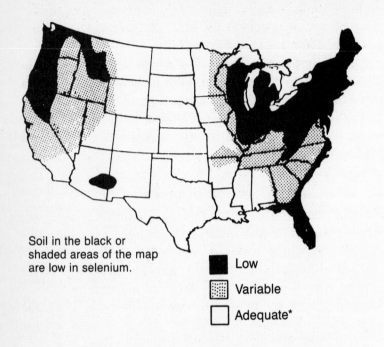

Soil in the black or
shaded areas of the map
are low in selenium.

■ Low

▨ Variable

☐ Adequate*

*In some areas identified as "adequate," agronomists fear that repeated
harvest of crops may be depleting the selenium which is not replaced.

FIGURE 10.

more effective in raising blood selenium levels than comparable
amounts of inorganic selenium salts.

All normal nutritional sources of selenium are organic in
form, consisting primarily of L-selenomethionine and, to a
lesser extent, other amino acids that contain selenium. Selenomethionine is selenium bound to the amino acid methionine.
The less desirable inorganic forms of selenium are sodium
selenite and sodium selenate.

Inorganic selenium compounds are normally absent in human

foods and have never been in the human food chain. Experiments have shown that they are metabolized differently than the natural organic dietary selenium sources. Selenomethionine is actively transported across the intestinal wall[7], whereas the selenite form is absorbed like a foreign or toxic substance.[8]

Selenomethionine is retained well in the body and evenly transported into tissues and organs, but the selenite and selenate forms tend to accumulate primarily in the liver and the kidneys. They are then excreted more rapidly.

Inorganic selenium salts (sodium selenite or sodium selenate) have to be taken in dosages that are much larger than the dosages needed with the organic selenium compounds in order to raise blood selenium levels effectively. Only products containing biologically incorporated or organically bound selenium are recommended for human supplementation.[9]

Nutrition 21, a research firm based in La Jolla, California, pioneered the process of growing yeast in a selenium-rich nutrient medium. These were the first good organically bound selenium products that were commercially available for human use.

Yeast is a nutritious food that has been in the human food supply for thousands of years. However, some people have trouble digesting yeast products properly. To meet the needs of yeast-sensitive individuals, Nutrition 21 has introduced recently a yeast-free L-selenomethionine product. They supply these products to the companies that make nutritional supplements and to the scientific community for research purposes. Both of these products are guaranteed to be free of *Candida albicans*, a different form of yeast that can cause difficulties in sensitive individuals.

Dosage Range

The FDA has set the recommended dietary intake of selenium at a range of 50 to 200 micrograms daily. Many scientists and nutritionists feel that the recommended daily intake should be raised to the level of 250–350 micrograms daily.

There is still some disagreement on the levels of selenium intake and supplementation for optimal health. According to Dr. Richard Passwater, a good compromise is to eat a well-balanced diet that provides 100 to 150 micrograms of selenium and then to take 100 to 200 micrograms of selenium daily as a supplement.[10] Our requirement for selenium increases under increased exposure to toxins and stress, just as do many other nutritional requirements.

According to Dr. Schrauzer, the evidence that selenium protects against cancer is strong enough to justify advising almost everyone to take from 250 to 300 micrograms of selenium as a daily supplement.[11]

Deficiency Symptoms

Selenium's primary function is that of a protector rather than a nutritional building block in our system. Therefore, deficiency symptoms are likely to be the beginnings of diseases that occur gradually over time with the continued destruction and aging of the body. Some of the symptoms reported are a depressed immune system, growth impairment, the development of cataracts, muscular dystrophy, liver problems, sterility (in males), heart disease, and cancer.

Side Effects and Toxicity

Selenium was neglected and overlooked in nutritional research for a long time because of its known toxicity at high levels.

Selenium is definitely toxic if excessive levels are ingested. The toxic level in humans is reported by the National Research Council to occur after long-term consumption of 2400 to 3000 micrograms daily. The toxic range is about one hundred times above the lowest effective nutritional dose. Inorganic selenium supplements such as sodium selenite are about three times more toxic than high-selenium yeast supplements.

The symptoms of selenium toxicity include loss of hair, nails, and teeth, skin inflammation, lassitude, paralysis, and eventual death. However, selenium toxicity in man is very rare because selenium compounds are readily excreted from the body, thus reducing the possibility of toxicity unless relatively large amounts are ingested on a regular basis. The real danger with selenium is its deficiency, not its toxicity.

Final Comments

Volumes of research now indicate that low blood selenium levels are associated with increased risks to cancer, heart disease, and a lowered immune system. After studying the United States dietary intakes of selenium, Dr. Gerhard Schrauzer, has suggested that doubling the current U.S. per capita selenium intake to about 250 to 300 mcg per day would utilize more fully selenium's protective capacity against the killer diseases. These levels of dietary selenium intake could be reached only by making major changes in present standard American diet (SAD diet). Also, selenium-rich foods would have to be transported into regions where selenium soil content is low. I do not expect to see these changes happen quickly. Therefore, daily dietary supplementation is the only reliable way to improve selenium status.

In summary, population studies, laboratory experiments, and clinical trials with selenium all come to similar conclusions. This research establishes without a doubt that selenium plays a vital role in the removal of toxic metals from our brain tissue, and in the prevention of heart disease and many forms of cancer. Proper use of selenium can also strengthen the body's immune system, improve energy levels, and slow the aging process.

23

Vitamin E: The Great Protector

Vitamin E is important to the maintenance of good mental functioning because it protects the cells of the brain as well as those of the entire body. This vitamin resides in the cell membrane, keeping the cell wall from being damaged. It prevents destruction of the neurons by blocking the action of free radicals.

Vitamin E can keep you looking younger by retarding cellular aging. A powerful antioxidant, vitamin E quenches free radicals that rob you of your youthful vitality and appearance. Vitamin E has many other health-promoting and antiaging properties that make it critical to optimal health and wellness.

Other important attributes of vitamin E are its ability to heal burns and prevent scarring, enhance the immune system, protect against cardiovascular diseases, and help prevent blood clots. In women, it helps prevent fibrocystic breast disease, and relieves symptoms of menopause. In conjunction with vitamin A, vitamin E protects against very damaging air pollutants, specifically nitrogen oxides and ozone. These two vitamins also work well together in protecting your skin from the sun's ultraviolet rays.

Vitamin E is actually the name of a family of chemicals called tocopherols. Nature produces eight different forms of tocopherol (named alpha, beta, gamma, delta, epsilon, zeta,

eta, and theta). Alpha-tocopherol has the widest natural distribution and the greatest biological activity.

Vitamin E is classified as a fat-soluble vitamin. By definition, a vitamin is an essential nutrient that causes a deficiency disease when it is absent from the diet. Because low levels of vitamin E do not produce well-defined vitamin deficiency diseases, the question of whether or not vitamin E is an essential nutrient has been a point of controversy for years. This argument misses the mark. Vitamin E does not function as a nutritional building block; it is a multipurpose defense mechanism against free radical damage.

Vitamin E, the great protector of our bodies, has two major metabolic roles:

1. It acts as nature's most potent fat-soluble antioxidant, protecting cellular membranes and the tiny structures inside the cell from damage. The high fat-containing cells of the brain, nervous system, and skin get their primary protection from vitamin E.[1]

2. It plays a role in selenium metabolism. Vitamin E and selenium seem to function as powerful antioxidant partners. They work together to neutralize several different types of free radicals and their synergistic activity is a fairly recent discovery. It has been reported that vitamin E is significantly more effective in the presence of selenium.[2]

Vitamin E's ability to protect unsaturated fats against oxidative damage is its most significant biological function; it is nature's best fat-soluble antioxidant.[3] Many other beneficial effects are a result of its role as an antioxidant.

Vitamin E and Heart Disease

There is an inverse relationship between the declining amount of vitamin E in the diet and the rising rate of heart attacks in the United States. In the last eighty years the average daily intake of vitamin E in our diets has gone from 150 IU to 7.4 IU.[4] Our modern methods of processing wheat and oils are responsible for the removal of vitamin E from our diets.

Vitamin E's protective or therapeutic effects in heart disease are still an area of controversy since there is not a large body of research that substantiates the claims. However, scientists know that vitamin E does reduce the platelet stickiness that helps prevent blood clotting and atherosclerosis.

Vitamin E and Your Brain

The cells in the brain and skin have a higher percentage of fat than the other cells in your body. The fats in these tissues are primarily the highly unsaturated essential fatty acids that are so easily oxidized. Vitamin E is the primary antioxidant that protects these cells from free radical attack, damage, and aging.

Vitamin E and Sex

Vitamin E has developed a reputation for being able to increase potency and virility. How did this reputation evolve? Tocopherol (vitamin E) is a Greek word that means "to bear children." The discoverer of tocopherol found that male rats deficient in vitamin E were sterile. Female rats deficient in vitamin E were unable to conceive. The inability to reproduce was corrected when the animals were given adequate vitamin E in their diets. This gave vitamin E the reputation as the "fertility vitamin," which led people to believe that it would enhance sexual prowess.

This is a misconception that occurred because vitamin E's discovery was associated with sperm potency in males and reproductive capability in females. Vitamin E is found in high concentration in the sex glands and it is vital for good functioning. This does not necessarily mean that it will increase potency and sexual drive. However, it has been reported that vitamin E can increase endurance, vitality, and well-being, which can indirectly increase sexual desire and activity.

Food Sources

The highest concentration of vitamin E is found in the oils of
nuts, seeds, and soybeans. These oils must be cold-pressed and
unrefined; there is almost no vitamin E in the refined oils
normally found in supermarkets. Soybeans, fresh wheat germ,
wheat germ oil, whole grains, eggs, nuts, and seeds are also
high in vitamin E. Smaller concentrations of vitamin E are
contained in dark leafy vegetables, brussels sprouts, broccoli,
cabbage, and asparagus.

Supplements

Vitamin E supplements can be purchased as: (1) natural mixed
tocopherols; (2) natural vitamin E (D-alpha-tocopherol); (3)
synthetic vitamin E (DL-alpha-tocopherol); (4) mycelized vitamin E.

Since nature makes eight different forms of vitamin E, we
may eventually find that each serves a purpose. Presently there
are no facts to support this reasoning other than the knowledge
that each form is absorbed differently, and they remain in the
body for different lengths of time. Some health professionals
suggest alternating back and forth between natural mixed
tocopherols and natural D-alpha-tocopherol.

Natural vs. Synthetic

An unsettled controversy still exists regarding natural versus
synthetic vitamin E supplements. Vitamin E, like many bio-
chemicals, can exist in two mirror-image forms. The right-
handed form is called "d-tocopherol" and the left-handed form
is called "l-tocopherol." When vitamin E is produced in nature,
it occurs in the "d" configuration only. Therefore, natural
vitamin E is written as d-alpha-tocopherol. When vitamin E is
prepared synthetically, it is a mixture of the "d" and "l" forms
and synthetic vitamin E is written as dl-alpha-tocopherol.

The biological potency of vitamin E preparations is expressed in terms of International Units (IU) of activity. Theoretically, 400 IU of synthetic vitamin E should have the same potency as 400 IU of natural vitamin E. It should not make any difference whether natural or synthetic vitamin E supplements are taken. However, this is not the case. Recent work by several researchers has shown that synthetic vitamin E has between 30 and 50 percent less biological activity than natural vitamin E.[5]

Dosage Range

Vitamin E is usually supplied in strengths ranging from 100 IU to 1000 IU (IU = International Units). It is available in oil-base capsules as well as water-soluble dry-base tablets. Natural vitamin E is approximately twice as expensive, but because of its greater biological potency, it is worth the price.

The government RDA for Vitamin E is 15 IU daily. Most nutritionally-oriented health professionals feel this is far below the level necessary for optimal health and nutrition. They often recommend that an average daily dosage range for high-level wellness is from 400 IU to 800 IU of natural vitamin E daily for adults.[6,7]

Absorption

Most people assume that whatever nutrients they take will be absorbed and made available to the body. This is not always true, especially with the fat-soluble vitamins. Vitamin E is a fat-soluble vitamin and therefore, it is not soluble in the water medium of the small intestine. The body must break down fats and fat-soluble vitamins in the intestine into very small particles in order for absorption to take place. People who do not accomplish this metabolic transformation efficiently will tend to suffer from malabsorption.

Mycelization

Mycelization is a fairly recent breakthrough in nutritional technology. In this process fat-soluble vitamins (E and A) are broken up into small particles so that they become water-soluble. This process dramatically increases the body's absorption of these vitamins and increases their incorporation into cellular membranes.

Mycelization provides much higher absorption, and therefore greater nutritional benefit. The bioavailability of the Mycelized supplement is two to five times greater than with the other forms of the vitamin.[8]

Several companies are marketing mycelized vitamin E now. Some of the mycelized products are made from natural vitamin E (d-alpha-tocopherol) and others are made from synthetic vitamin E (dl-alpha-tocopherol). High-quality mycelized vitamin products (made from natural vitamin E) can be purchased in health food stores.

Mycelized Vitamin E is sold in 1 oz. bottles with a 1 ml dropper. Its potency is: 1 ml of mycelized vitamin E = 150 IU. This is equivalent to 720 IU of oil E or 330 IU of emulsified E. Using a daily dose of half a dropper (equivalent to 400 IU of the old unmycelized form), one bottle will last about two months.

Deficiency Symptoms

Deficiency symptoms for vitamin E are restlessness, fatigue, menopausal symptoms, fitful sleep, and insomnia. Severe deficiency results in increased destruction of red blood cells, muscle wasting, increased demand for oxygen, poor glandular function, and liver and kidney damage.

Vitamin Robbers

Vitamin E supplements are important especially for the millions of women who regularly take birth control pills. Research shows that oral contraceptives lower the blood level of vitamin E, which increases the individual's dietary requirement for it.[9]

Chlorine is an environmental toxin that destroys vitamin E. The most common exposure to chlorine is in cities where it is added to the municipal drinking water. You may want to consider investing in a water purification unit or buying a good brand of bottled water.

Malabsorption is another problem that robs people of vitamin E. Taking the nutrient orally does not mean that it is being absorbed into your system. This is a problem that increases with age, and consequently, it is frequently a problem in the elderly. However, the mycelized vitamins mentioned earlier are easily absorbed, even by people with absorption problems.

Side Effects and Toxicity

The most common complaints following inappropriately large doses of vitamin E are gastrointestinal disturbances including nausea, gas, or diarrhea.[10] However, because vitamin E is essentially nontoxic, these side effects are seldom seen. Vitamin E is a fat-soluble vitamin. Any fat-soluble vitamin has the potential to be absorbed in the tissues and to be toxic at excessively high levels. However, the toxicity scare with vitamin E has been blown far out of proportion. Unlike other fat-soluble vitamins, vitamin E is stored in the body for a relatively short time; from 60 to 70 percent of the daily dose is excreted in the feces.

To double the blood content of vitamin E, the dosage must be increased by a factor of forty. Increasing the consumption of vitamin E from 100 IU to 500 IU only increased the blood level of vitamin E by 9 percent.[11] However, there is some evidence that doses above 1000 IU daily can suppress the immune system.[12]

Contraindications

Individuals with rheumatic heart disease, severe heart failure, or excessively high blood pressure should not take more than 200 IU of vitamin E daily without being under the supervision of a physician. People with these problems should take the water-soluble or mycelized forms of vitamin E rather than the oil forms.

Final Comments

Without a doubt, everyone should take supplemental E and selenium for the benefits they provide. However, what is really needed is an increase in the public's overall nutritional awareness. The emphasis should be not only on individual vitamins, but on the necessity of optimal, balanced levels of all nutrients. Vitamin E is one of the strongest players on your nutritional team, but it can't play alone.

24
Vitamin A/Beta-Carotene: Preserving Intelligence

Vitamin A is important to the preservation of intelligence because of its function as a fat-soluble antioxidant. As a protector of brain cells the effects of Vitamin A are not evident, since we do not notice what we have and have not lost. Besides preventing damage to neurons, A and beta-carotene can promise you soft, smooth skin for a lifetime. These powerful antioxidant nutrients are becoming famous as major anticancer nutrients as well. Vitamin A and beta-carotene are youth-restoring vitamins.

Vitamin A is a fat-soluble antioxidant vitamin that exists in two different forms:

1. Vitamin A (also called retinol), found only in foods from animal sources in its pre-formed state.

2. Beta-carotene (also called pro-vitamin A), found primarily in plant food sources.

Beta-carotene is converted by the body into vitamin A. It is an excellent source of vitamin A because an enzyme in the liver splits one molecule of beta-carotene in half, producing two molecules of vitamin A.

Effects

Vitamin A and beta-carotene are fat-soluble antioxidant nutrients. This means they reside in, are stored in, and protect tissues in the body that contain high concentrations of fat in their cellular structure. You will recall that the highest fat-containing tissues needing these types of protection are the brain and the skin. Fats are primary components of cellular membranes, and they are the components that are most easily damaged. Therefore, it is one of vitamin A's primary functions to protect cell membranes.

Vitamin A promotes the growth of healthy skin, hair, and nails. It is vital in the treatment of acne and many other types of skin conditions. It also protects the skin from the cancer causing ultraviolet rays from the sun. Good vision, particularly night vision, is another benefit of proper vitamin A intake. Vitamin A also stimulates the immune system. It protects against infections and it speeds up the healing process.

There is overwhelming evidence accumulating that demonstrates the role of Vitamin A and beta-carotene in the prevention of numerous types of cancer in humans. Recent studies seem to indicate that beta-carotene is the more powerful anticancer agent. Population studies show that people who have lower levels of beta-carotene in their diet have a higher incidence of many types of cancer.[1]

Beta-carotene—Special Properties

Beta-carotene has some unique properties of its own, independent of its function as a precursor of vitamin A. It is a powerful antioxidant that neutralizes two of the most damaging free radicals—polyunsaturated fatty acid radicals and the singlet oxygen free radical.

The toxicity of oxygen free radicals is considered to be a primary factor in chronic degenerative diseases and aging. The singlet oxygen free radical is one of the most damaging of the oxygen radicals. It is formed during regular metabolic processes, and also as a result of exposure to direct sunlight (ultraviolet rays) or ozone. Our bodies have specific antioxidant enzymes to deal with many of the other free radicals, but we have not developed an enzyme to neutralize the singlet oxygen radical. This is why beta-carotene is of such importance. *It is the only substance that can quench the oxygen radical and prevent the destruction it can do.*[2]

Food Sources

Vitamin A concentrates in the liver. Therefore, high levels of vitamin A can be obtained from beef, chicken, fish liver, or fish liver oils. Plant sources high in beta-carotene are carrots, spinach, swiss chard, collard greens, kale, broccoli, sweet potatoes, winter squash, pumpkin, apricots, cantaloupes, and papaya.

Supplements

Vitamin A is available as a dietary supplement in health food stores and the vitamin section of many retail drug stores. The most common form of vitamin A is derived from fish liver oil. This form is usually packaged in gelatin capsules containing 10,000 IU or 25,000 IU.

Beta-carotene is available in capsule or powder form. The bulk powder is more economical, but messy to work with. Microscopic amounts of beta-carotene "dust" can create a bright orange kitchen counter.

Vitamin A has become available recently in the mycelized form. Mycelized vitamin A is available in liquid form in 1 oz. bottles with a 1 ml dropper. One drop of liquid contains 5000 IU. Because of the greater degree of absorption, this form is over five times as effective as the common oil-based vitamin A supplement: 1 drop (5000 IU) = 27,000 units oil A.

Using a daily dose of one or two drops of mycelized A, a single bottle will last almost a year. This is more cost effective than the traditional forms of vitamin A supplementation. Mycelized vitamin supplements are carried in most good health food stores now.

Since beta-carotene is a nontoxic precursor to vitamin A and has special antioxidant properties of its own, many health professionals are recommending a high ratio of beta-carotene to vitamin A. Beta-carotene can be converted into vitamin A if storage of vitamin A is deficient.

Dosage Range

The RDA for vitamin A is 5000 IU daily. The dosage range recommended by many health professionals for high-level wellness is from 10,000 to 35,000 IU daily. People with individual special needs and/or people with poor health habits (such as smoking) may require much higher levels for optimal protection and health.

The liver is the primary storage site for vitamin A in our bodies. Mobilizing vitamin A from the liver storage sites requires adequate dietary zinc. A daily multi-mineral supplement that contains 20–25 mg of zinc is regarded by many health professionals as normally sufficient.

The dosages for infants and children are substantially lower than adult levels, depending on weight, age, and individual health. Consult with a qualified health professional before giving a child or infant vitamin A supplements. Cod liver oil is a good source of vitamin A for children and it is available in mint and cherry flavors.

Vitamin A and beta-carotene are absorbed more completely if taken with a fat-containing meal. Gastrointestinal or liver diseases inhibit the body from absorbing vitamin A. People with gall bladder disturbances and diabetics may also be poor absorbers of vitamin A and beta-carotene. People with these problems may require much higher dosage levels of fat-soluble vitamins, but only under the guidance of a qualified health professional.

Deficiency Symptoms

When there is a deficiency of vitamin A, the mucous membranes become impaired. This can lead to any of the following deficiency symptoms of vitamin A: acne, dry scaly skin, peeling nails, dandruff, low luster hair, frequent respiratory infections, and precancerous changes in body tissue. Other key deficiency symptoms are related to vision, such as night blindness and tired, achy eyes.

Vitamin A can be depleted by stress, air pollutants, antacids, aspirin, barbiturates, and several types of prescription drugs.

Side Effects and Toxicity

Taking too much beta-carotene can lead to an interesting (and harmless) effect called kerotenosis. This is a temporary, yellow-orange discoloration of the skin that is most easily seen on the palms of the hand and soles of the feet. Simply decreasing the dosage will cause this coloring to disappear.

Since vitamin A is a fat-soluble vitamin, excesses are stored in the body and can result in toxicity. However, the fear of vitamin A toxicity has been somewhat exaggerated. There is a wide range between the maximum physiological requirement and the amount necessary to cause toxicity. Vitamin A toxicity results only when very large quantities are taken.

Toxicity signs for vitamin A include dry, rough skin, a yellowing of both the skin and whites of the eyes, painful joint swellings, nausea, headaches, fatigue, enlarged liver, and irregular menses. These symptoms quickly disappear after the dosage is normalized. It is also reported that these symptoms can be prevented by taking generous amounts of vitamin C.[3]

The situation with beta-carotene is quite different. Cells in the small intestine and in the liver convert beta-carotene into usable vitamin A. However, this conversion only takes place when the body is in need of vitamin A. As a result, vitamin A toxicity *cannot* result from ingesting beta-carotene.

Final Comments

A study published in the *American Journal of Clinical Nutrition* examined the dietary habits of both poor and upper income people and found that possibly as many as 37 percent of Americans are not getting enough vitamin A. To put it another way, over one third of our entire population is in the "poor risk" group with regard to vitamin A.

The only raw materials your body has from which to manufacture good health are the foods and nutrients that you put into it. Vitamin A and beta-carotene are key players in the creation and maintenance of good health throughout your life.

25

Gerovital/GH-3: "The Amazing Rejuvenation Formula"

Gerovital or GH-3 is the most famous and the most popular antiaging therapy of all time. It has been called the "youth drug" and the "amazing rejuvenation formula." Some studies have concluded that it has amazing powers to restore mental and physical health. Other studies conclude that it has a clear effect as an antidepressant but no other proven therapeutic benefits. We will review these studies in this chapter so you can evaluate the conflicting evidence for yourself.

Gerovital was developed by Dr. Ana Aslan, director of the Institute for Geriatrics in Bucharest, Romania. She announced the availability of this new, effective antiaging drug at a medical conference in September 1956. GH-3 has been an issue of debate and controversy ever since it first became available.

Is Gerovital an antiaging breakthrough or is it a hoax? Does it deserve its fame or is it a fraud? This chapter will attempt to shed some light on these questions.

Gerovital/Procaine

Gerovital is a 2 percent procaine hydrochloride solution. It also contains trace amounts of benzoic acid, potassium metabisulfate, and disodium phosphate that act as buffers or stabilizers.

The biologically active ingredient in Gerovital is procaine. Procaine hydrochloride by itself is a product that is used frequently by dentists. It is a local anesthetic that is marketed under the trade name Novacaine. However, you do not get numb when you take gerovital orally or by injection.

In the body, procaine is broken down into two metabolites, para-aminobenzoic acid (PABA) and diethyl-aminoethanol (DEAE). PABA is a lesser-known member of the B-vitamins. The DEAE half of procaine is structurally a very close relative of DMAE (see Chapter 8). A prescription drug named Thorazine (chlorpromazine) contains DEAE as part of its structure.[1]

Benefits of Gerovital

The advertisements for GH-3 claim that research throughout the world has "demonstrated the effectiveness of GH-3 therapy for more than 200 diseases and ailments related to premature aging." They list the following:

Senility	Hypertension
Arthritis	Sexual impotence
Gray hair & balding	Insomnia
Wrinkling skin	Heart disease
Stress	Hormonal deficiencies
Depression	Angina pectoris
Fatigue	Poor hearing
Liver or age spots	Alzheimer's disease
Parkinson's disease	Migraine headache
Poor circulation	Liver disease
Alcoholism	Chronic pain
Poor memory	Lung disease[2]

As you can see, this is quite a list of apparent benefits. One of the problems associated with Gerovital is the lack of professionalism and the sensationalism in the efforts to market the drug. The marketing of this drug even goes to the extent that the government of Romania has advertised "package deals" and special flights inviting people to come to Romania for Dr. Ana Aslan's original GH-3 therapy.

Effects of Gerovital

Life extension. Antiaging and rejuvenation head the list of claims made for Gerovital. In one of Dr. Aslan's early studies, she reported that Gerovital increased the life span of male rats by 21.2 percent and of females by 6.7 percent.[3]

An Austrian study that attempted to duplicate the life extension results reported by Aslan was unsuccessful. However, this study administered very high doses of the drug, which may have produced some overriding toxic effects.[4]

However, the Texas Research Institute for Mental Sciences reported that mice receiving Gerovital had a 33 percent higher survival rate at the end of the study (twenty-five months of age) than controls. This study also showed that the Gerovital brains of the GH-3 treated mice had a more stabilized cell membrane function relative to the usual deterioration of membranes in normal untreated animals.[5]

In 1957 Dr. Aslan published results of a large human trial involving over five thousand patients. In this paper she described case histories with dramatic improvements in both physical and mental function.[6]

During the early 1960s a number of studies were conducted in England and the United States in an attempt to try to duplicate the claims of Gerovital on aging made by Dr. Aslan. Over a period of several years, eight well-controlled double-blind studies testing procaine on aging were published.

A summary of those reports shows that six studies reported no benefits for the procaine-treated patients over controls; the other two reported slight benefits in psychologic and cognitive functions for the procaine-treated patients.[7]

There are actually two controversies that have developed over the years relating to the claims and testing of Gerovital. The first is the Gerovital vs. procaine argument. Dr. Aslan points out that the studies attempting to duplicate her findings are using only procaine hydrochloride, with no additives. She states that the buffers and stabilizers in her Gerovital formulation are essential to its effectiveness. Other scientists point out that these claims are only speculations that have never been tested or proven scientifically.

The second half of the controversy centers on those scientists who have criticized Dr. Aslan's published studies on Gerovital. They claim that her research studies are not well designed or controlled, and cannot be duplicated.

Observations during early clinical trials with Gerovital lead researchers to believe that some of the changes and improvements seen in patients were the result of the relief of depression. Subsequent pharmacological studies showed that procaine could affect a change in brain chemistry that could relieve certain states of depression. Thus it became apparent that some of the original improvements that were labeled rejuvenation and antiaging were really the result of an antidepressant effect.

Depression. Gerovital's ability to act as an antidepressant is another primary claim and one that has more scientifically supportive documentation. Some researchers have shown that Gerovital inhibits an enzyme called monoamine oxidase (MAO).[8] In the pharmaceutical industry a major class of antidepressants are called MAO inhibitors. These are powerful drugs that have significant side effects associated with them. Gerovital avoids these side effects because it acts as a weak, reversible MAO inhibitor.

Several well-controlled, double-blind studies have documented Gerovital's effectiveness as an antidepressant in people over fifty. A study on depression at Duke University compared Gerovital with Tofranil (generic name imipramine). Tofranil is a prescription drug that is commonly prescribed for depression. They found that Gerovital was significantly more effective than Tofranil in treating depression.[9]

Another study on aging patients with depression reported that patients, "felt a greater sense of well-being and relaxation, slept better at night, and many obtained some relief from depression and the discomforts of chronic inflammation or degenerative disease."[10]

On the other side, Dr. Israel Zwerling, from the Bronx Hospital in New York, concluded in his study that Gerovital was "not effective" in treating depression.[11] Researchers in the Brentwood V.A. Hospital in Los Angeles, concluded that the drug was no better than a placebo.[12] Yet another study done by James Clemens of the Eli Lilly company indicated only a slight inhibition of MAO in rats at much higher doses than humans would consume. He concluded that, if GH-3 was an effective antidepressant in a clinic setting, it was probably not due to MAO inhibition.[13]

Critics of Dr. Aslan's clinical studies point out another problem in her studies associated with depression. It is known that depression can cause a treatable form of dementia. Some of Dr. Aslan's critics say that she took lonely, elderly people from the dull, dreary atmosphere of Romanian retirement homes, and moved them to her institute's pleasant environment where they were given Gerovital *and* personal attention. Certainly changes of this nature could subsequently be responsible for less depression and result in improvements in some of the symptoms of aging.[14]

Memory. Claims for Gerovital also indicate that it can be helpful for individuals suffering from poor memory and senility. A study published in 1984 gives a possible explanation for these effects. This study documented procaine's ability to improve the brain's ability to utilize oxygen. Procaine improved the oxygen utilization in old rats to levels that were equal to those in young rats. The authors of this study state that procaine increased the levels of respiratory enzymes, which in turn increases oxygen consumption and energy levels in the brain.[15]

Gerovital Reviewed

A major review of the world literature on procaine/Gerovital was published in the *Journal of the American Geriatrics Society*, January 1977. This review correlated data from twenty-five years of procaine therapy on over 100,000 patients. The authors state that,

> Except for a possible antidepressant effect, there is no convincing evidence that procaine (or Gerovital, of which procaine is the major component) has any value in the treatment of disease in older patients. If procaine has an antidepressant effect, there is some likelihood that this accounts for the reports of decreased complaints referable to the musculoskeletal, cardiovascular, endocrine, sexual, gastrointestinal, and respiratory systems.[16]

A more recent review of the literature (1983) concluded by saying, "there is no convincing evidence to support any of the claims made for procaine in treatment of the aged, with the possible exception of an antidepressant effect and, perhaps, an improvement in mental acuity."[17]

Yet numerous clinical trials published in the professional literature report that Gerovital does produce beneficial results. In addition to improvements in mental condition, improvements of general physical condition in patients are also reported.[18]

As you can see, the history of GH-3 is one of controversy and questions. There has always been a tremendous amount of media attention and sensationalism surrounding GH-3. Movie stars, heads of government, kings and queens have rushed to Romania to be treated by Dr. Aslan. Many people purchase GH-3 based on its advertising claims. They are willing to try a new "miracle drug" because they are dissatisfied with the options and results that conventional medicine has to offer.

Dosage

Oral. In oral form, one GH-3 tablet is taken daily for twenty-five days. Then rest for five days before beginning another round.

Injectable. When injectable therapy is used, one injection is given every third day for thirty days. Then rest one month before doing another series of the injections.[19]

Side Effects

There are no reports of serious, acute, or chronic reactions in the use of Gerovital. However, a Russian report does caution against using procaine therapy indiscriminately in the elderly, especially in patients with advanced cardiovascular disease and/or hypertension.

Availability

Gerovital is available as a nonprescription drug in Romania as well as other European countries, and in Mexico. It has never been approved by the Food and Drug Administration (FDA) in the United States. However, in 1977 the state of Nevada passed a bill making Gerovital legally available. It can be dispensed only by a licensed pharmacist but does not require a prescription. It does require, however, that the buyer sign for it.

For information about Gerovital you may contact the Romanian National Tourist Office, 573 Third Avenue, New York, NY 10016. Their phone is (212) 697-6971.

Gerovital (GH-3) is also available from Pharmaceuticals International, 539 Telegraph Canyon Road, Suite 227, Chula Vista, CA 92010-6492.

Summary

When Dr. Ana Aslan introduced GH-3 to the world in 1956 as an important new antiaging compound, her findings were met with broadscale skepticism. Yet today it has become one of the most, if not the most, popular rejuvenation product in the world. Thousands of people report benefits from its use. Many people believe that it is one of the safest and most effective long term antidepressants known.

26

Exercise and the Mind

Exercise is the most powerful antiaging drug for your brain. The primary benefit of exercise is oxygenation, which decreases free radical damage throughout your body and especially in the brain, thus deterring the aging process. Exercise actually releases drug-like substances into the central nervous system such as endorphins, creating euphoria and eliminating depression. Another substance released is norepinephrine, which stimulates mental alertness and enhances memory.

Virtually everyone knows that exercise is important to health, but most people do not realize just how important it is for both mental and physical well-being. Why should we exercise and what are the benefits we gain from it? Not only does it improve physical health and endurance, it enables you to maintain that level of health into your later years. It also increases motivation and productivity while improving mood and attitude. In addition, it improves reaction time, levels of thinking and reasoning, and enhances short term memory and recall capabilities.

Exercise and the Aging Process

Do you know anyone at the age of sixty who looks seventy-five and feels seventy-five? Do you know anyone who is sixty years old and looks only forty-five and feels it? It is not uncommon to encounter elderly people who are lucid in their nineties and others who are senile at sixty-five. People like this are good examples of individuals whose chronological age does not match their biological age. What could be responsible for this? There could be a lot of reasons for the differences, but you can be sure that one of the biggest factors is exercise.

Dr. Walter Bortz, M.D., professor of medicine at Palo Alto Medical Clinic in California, investigated the relationship between exercise and aging in his paper called "Disuse and Aging." He found that the deterioration of the body caused by aging is often identical to the destruction caused by physical inactivity. Physical conditions often associated with age are a decrease in the body's supply of oxygen, decreased cardiac output, depressed immune system, lowered metabolic and regulatory functions, and decreased sexual function. These are often identical to conditions seen in sedentary individuals of any age.

Dr. Bortz suggests that changes and conditions commonly attributed to aging may be no more than symptoms of disuse or inactivity. In each case studied, Dr. Bortz reports that exercise could reverse the decline. He further cites animal studies that demonstrate that female and male rats that exercised lived 12 percent and 20 percent longer than their sedentary counterparts. In conclusion, Dr. Bortz states, "There is no drug in current or prospective use that holds as much promise for sustained health as a lifetime program of physical exercise."[1]

Exercise and Mental Energy

Imagine yourself next to a powerful waterfall that has tremendous force and movement. How does it feel? You most likely feel energized, vibrant, and relaxed all at the same time. Now imagine yourself next to a stagnant pond. Do you experience the same feeling? Probably not. *Movement creates energy.* The movement of the waterfall can produce electricity and power. A stagnant pond invites pests and potential malignant growth. The same analogy applies to exercising your mind and body.

Exercise increases blood circulation to the brain, which makes more oxygen available to the cells. This translates into more mental energy. Exercise helps create a bright, alert, clear-thinking mind, a strong sense of well-being, and the energy to accomplish tasks.

A common excuse many people use for not exercising is that they do not have enough energy to exercise. Ironically, the opposite is true. These people do not have any energy *because* they do not exercise. It is highly likely that their energy will not improve until they begin to exercise.

No doubt we have all had the experience of simply not feeling like moving after a demanding day of work. It is at this point that you will gain the most from movement. Have you ever heard anyone after a good workout say they wished they had not exercised? I never have. That is because the stresses of the day have been released, an increased amount of oxygen has been delivered to the cells, and the mind and body are energized.

There is more involved in this experience of greater mental and physical energy resulting from exercise than just a subjective feeling. There is actually a change that takes place in your brain cells.

When you exercise on a regular basis, you actually increase your cellular metabolism. Inside our cells are little organelles called mitochondria. An organelle is a small organ inside a cell. There are many mitochondria inside each cell. The job of the mitochondria is to turn food into energy. They are, in essence, tiny energy-producing power plants inside our cells. We derive our energy from the energy output of the mitochondria.

When we exercise we increase the efficiency of the inner workings of the mitochondria. When we supply them with optimal oxygen, they are more able to fully convert food into energy. Complete metabolism decreases the amount of waste material and toxic buildup. We therefore gain full benefit from our nutrients, and our cells accumulate fewer toxins.

Exercise also causes the mitochondria to work harder, generating more energy. This is the connection between exercise and your energy level. The more we require of the mitochondria, the stronger they get. There is even more to this story. When you exercise regularly and create a frequent demand for more energy, more mitochondrial energy factories are created in each cell. Exercise also makes existing mitochondria become larger in size. They therefore produce more energy on a constant basis.

Good mental functioning is directly related to one's energy levels. Those who exercise on a regular basis have stronger mitochondrial energy factories working for them on a constant basis, providing a solid energy base for clear thinking, problem solving, synthesizing information, and memory retention. The result of these positive mental changes is an alert mind.

Exercise and the Mind

The body of research studying the relationship of exercise to the brain and mental functioning is growing rapidly. Researchers are discovering that mental alertness, intelligence, and the prevention of senility are directly related to one's level of exercise. They also are beginning to understand the profound effect exercise has on moods, depression, and general mental health.

Exercise is an antidepressant. In a study of healthy subjects who exercised regularly, it was found that they experienced a positive mood immediately after a period of vigorous exercise and that the effects of these positive biochemical changes lasted for up to five hours after the exercise.[2] The release of endorphins, opiate-like brain chemicals that promote a sense of well-being and even euphoria, is one of reasons for this mood alteration. Other neurotransmitters that affect our moods, such as serotonin and norepinephrine, also undergo changes in response to exercise.

During a good aerobic workout, the heart will pump five times more oxygenated blood throughout your system, most of which is diverted to your muscles. During the same workout, the supply of oxygenated blood to the brain doubles. Conversely, there is a decrease in blood flow to the brain during depression.

Dr. Robert S. Brown, Ph.D., M.D., from the University of Virginia, has experimented extensively with various types of physical exercise to give relief to the depressed patient. He notes, "The inertia that accompanies the depressed person's increasing tendency to withdraw, his constriction of interests and preoccupation with unhappiness makes it tempting to hypothesize that some of the features of depression may be symptoms of a primary movement disorder."[3]

Building and exercising your mental muscles will increase your mental capabilities and slow down brain aging. In a study done at the Salt Lake City V.A. hospital, Dr. Robert Dustman took two groups of out-of-shape people aged fifty-five to seventy and put them on a four-month program of various types and levels of exercise. He also monitored a control group of nonexercisers.

At the end of four months, tests showed that the subjects who exercised had improved reaction time, improved levels of thinking and reasoning, and also showed better short-term memory and recall capabilities. The control group showed no change. Of further interest, the exercise group that participated in aerobic activities, slow jogging, and fast walking improved significantly more than those who did only strength and flexibility exercises.

Dr. Dustman stated that he and his associates were surprised by the amount of improvement that exercise produced. They expected to see some results in a few people, but they did not think they would see improvements of such magnitude in all of the participants.[4] This experiment clearly demonstrates the importance of participating in regular aerobic exercise.

The intellectual capabilities of children also have been shown to increase from exercise. In a controlled study—the Trois Rivières experiment—primary school children who had one hour of physical activity per day received higher grades, performed better on regional evaluations, and had better physical perceptions and coordination. This study supports the theory of many developmental psychologists that exercise stimulates psychomotor development in children.[5]

Dr. Thaddeus Samorajski, in his report at the International Congress of Biomedical Gerontology Conference in 1985, discussed the relationship between exercise and the maintenance of intellect. He stated that just as lung capacity can be improved by exercise, so can intelligence and memory be improved by practice and training.

In his study with laboratory animals, Dr. Samorajski determined that exercise improved memory retention and increased the norepinephrine content of the brain. Norepinephrine is a key neurotransmitter involved with memory and learning. This neurotransmitter is also known to enhance mental acuity.[6]

It is becoming more and more evident that exercise is directly related to the brain neurotransmitters that regulate mental functions. In addition to regulating these important brain chemicals, exercise transports oxygen to the brain. Oxygen is critical to optimal brain functioning and the prevention of brain aging.

Exercise and Oxygen

Exercise provides more of the most important nutrient there is, oxygen. Oxygen is the most critical nutrient for health and wellness. Our bodies are actually combustion engines, and oxygen is the fuel that makes them run. Oxygen metabolizes our food and turns it into energy. However, not only is oxygen the great healer, it is also the great slayer. Why is that so and how does it relate to the place of exercise in developing a lifestyle for optimal health, wellness, and mental functioning?

Remember from our earlier discussions that several of the most damaging types of free radicals are the toxic forms of oxygen, such as singlet oxygen and superoxide. Oxygen is a unique substance because it can create free radicals, as well as quench or neutralize them. Investigators have found that the main damage from a lack of oxygen to any cell or tissue comes from the free radicals that are produced during oxygen deficiency.

When the oxygen supply to any cell or tissue is optimal, the rate of oxygen-free radical generation is about the same as the rate at which oxygen inhibits the formation of free radicals. However, whenever the oxygen supply drops below its optimal level, its ability to inhibit or quench free radicals decreases drastically.

An example of just how significant the damage can be when oxygen supply drops below its optimal levels is seen in stroke victims. A stroke victim will often suffer partial paralysis, a droopy face, and slurred speech. This happens when the oxygen supply has decreased or has been cut off during the stroke.

The damage from strokes and heart attacks are extreme examples of free radical damage due to a lack of oxygen. This is actually what is happening on a gradual scale during the aging process. When brain cells receive suboptimal levels of oxygen, they are continually exposed to more free radicals. This is why exercise is so important to health. It is the process of keeping the oxygen levels optimal that prevents or at least significantly slows down free radical damage and aging.

Exercise and the Cardiovascular System

During exercise you force the heart muscle to work. The heart is like any other muscle in that exercising makes it stronger and healthier. This in turn allows the heart to pump more blood and oxygen with each strong stroke. The healthy, exercised heart

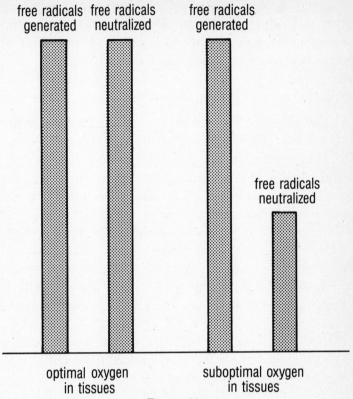

FIGURE 11.
The Difference Between the Amount of Free Radicals
Generated in Tissues When Oxygen Levels Are Optimal
Versus Suboptimal

pumps a greater volume of blood with each individual stroke. Therefore, it beats fewer times per minute and has a longer rest between strokes. The weaker heart muscle—in people who do not exercise—has to beat more times per minute to move the same volume of blood. Not only is the underexercised heart less efficient, it also has a shorter rest time between strokes. This is another reason why people who do not exercise fatigue more easily, both mentally and physically.

Now that we've discussed the cardiovascular system, blood supply, and oxygen as they relate to exercise, I think it is important to discuss a lesser known, yet equally important topic related to exercise and health, the lymphatic system.

The Lymphatic System

The lymphatic system is a series of vessels that lie parallel to the blood vessels and capillaries in the cardiovascular system. There is three times more lymph fluid than blood in the human body! Lymph fluid is not confined to the lymphatic vessels. It also surrounds and bathes every cell in the body. One of its functions is to bring nutrients from the blood to the cells. It also helps remove waste and toxins from the cells, functioning like the body's garbage disposal system.

The lymph is an integral part of the immune system. It carries the phagocytes and lymphocytes, which are the cells that surround and destroy viruses, bacteria, and other toxic substances.

The major difference between the cardiovascular system and the lymphatic system is the heart muscle. The cardiovascular system has this marvelous pump that forces the blood through the system of vessels. However, the lymphatic system has no such pump. It is a network of vessels and tubes with walls that are only one cell thick. The insides of the lymph vessels are lined with one-way valves.

The contraction and relaxation of your muscles provides a pumping action that increases the efficiency of the lymphatic system. Also, the expansion and contraction of the chest cavity during deep breathing stimulates the lymphatics. Therefore, aerobic exercise is the most effective way to activate the lymphatic system. By increasing the flow of lymph we clean out the old fluid surrounding the cells and increase the ability of the lymph nodes to fight off disease. By increasing the health and well-being of the physical body, our mental activity is supported. The ancient saying, "A healthy mind in a healthy body" applies.

How Much and What Kind of Exercise?

The amount of exercise necessary to gain all the benefits we have discussed throughout this chapter is a topic subject to controversy. However, I advise people to follow a general aerobic standard used by many health professionals and exercise physiologists. They recommend twenty to thirty minutes of aerobic exercise, three to four days per week. It is important to begin the workout with a warm-up to get your heart rate up. Then, for at least twenty minutes, it is advisable to maintain your heart rate at 80 percent of its maximum rate. This will stress you to the point of breathing heavily, and it will probably make you sweat. For some people walking will be enough. A trained athlete will have to work much harder to get the appropriate benefit for his or her level. There are many good books on the market today that can give you more detailed information in the area of aerobic exercise.

It is not my intention to be prescriptive of the type of exercise to choose. I do, however, want to make you aware of the different classes and types of exercise. There are basically three main types of exercise: aerobic exercise, anaerobic exercise, and exercises that focus on flexibility and coordination. Aerobic exercise is physical exertion sustained over a long time, such as jogging or swimming. Anaerobic exercise involves high-intensity exertion for very short periods of time—like weight-lifting or sprinting. Yoga and tai chi are examples of exercises that emphasize flexibility and coordination.

Exercises that produce high aerobic intensity are running or jogging, cross-country skiing, jumping rope, running in place, cycling, and rowing. Exercises that produce a lower level of aerobic intensity are dancing, tennis, other racket sports, swimming, and walking.

The issue is not which form of exercise you pick. The issue is that you *do* some form of aerobic exercise on a regular basis. Just getting started is most of the battle. It is also important that you choose a type of exercise that is fun for you. Sometimes, exercising with a friend or partner adds to the enjoyment. Exercise is more effective when you have fun and are doing it because you really want to. Just remember how good you feel when you are done!

In summary, exercise is one of the most important practices you can adopt for maximal mental and physical functioning. It is a long-term commitment to mental alertness, full utilization of your mind, a strong body, and long, happy life. Dr. Bortz's powerful statement deserves repeating, "There is no drug in current or prospective use that holds as much promise for sustained health as a lifetime program of physical exercise."[7]

27

Fats and Oils and the Brain

Why is a book that focuses on intelligence and mental enhancement devoting a chapter to fats and oils? Because our brain cells are comprised of 60 percent fat. This represents the highest concentration of fat in cells found anywhere in the body. The types of fats in your body play a key role in the development and maintenance of a healthy brain. Damage to fats is at the core of biological aging.

How well you understand and utilize the information on fats will play a significant role in how long you live and utilize the intelligence you have. In order to aid in your understanding of this subject, it will be helpful to have a brief overview of nutrition.

"You are what you eat" may be a cliché, but it is true. The only raw materials your body has to manufacture good health are the ones you put into it. What are the "things" that a body needs for good health?

Scientists have determined that there are forty-five essential nutrients. An essential nutrient is one that is absolutely necessary for good health, and one that the body cannot make itself. Therefore, it must be provided through the diet. A lack of, or even a marginal deficiency in, any essential nutrient will eventually result in a deterioration of health, the manifestation of some form of chronic degenerative disease, and loss of brain function.

Nature does not make mistakes. If you give the body what it needs, it will work like the marvelous miracle that it is. If it is deprived of some of its essential nutrients, it will attempt to tell you what it needs through the signs and symptoms of disease, which are your body's messages that something is wrong.

Essential Nutrients

What are these essential nutrients we need to keep our minds and bodies happy and healthy? There are twenty minerals, fifteen vitamins, eight essential amino acids, and two essential fatty acids. For optimal health and wellness, we need optimal quantities of every one of these forty-five essential nutrients.

The two essential fatty acids are the nutrients we need the most on a daily basis. These fats are referred to as Omega-3 (alpha-linolenic acid) and Omega-6 (linoleic acid). The body uses these two essential fatty acids to produce other necessary fatty acids. Thus you will sometimes hear about the Omega-3 and Omega-6 families of essential fatty acids.[1]

An Omega-3 international conference held in Italy in 1988 has settled on a new name for Omega-3. In the future you will be seeing it referred to as Alena, which is an acronym from Alpha-linolenic acid.

Although some individuals may be deficient in both essential fatty acids, the greatest nutritional deficiency in the average American diet is the lack of the Omega-3 (alpha-linolenic acid). One of the essential nutrients we need the most is the one we are the most deficient in!

The important thing to remember is that essential fatty acid deficiency is one of the primary causes of chronic degenerative disease. A loss of these essential nutrients in our diets has resulted in a steady increase in the incidence of the major diseases of our time, i.e., cancer, cardiovascular disease, diabetes, arthritis, high blood pressure, and strokes.

There are three basic reasons why the important essential

fatty acids have been almost nonexistent in our food supply. They are:

1. The milling of grain to produce white flour.
2. Eating beef as the primary source of protein.
3. The processing and hydrogenation of vegetable oils.[2]

Of these three, it is my opinion that the processing and hydrogenation of commercial oils is the most serious problem. The milling of the flour removes essential fats and ingesting beef provides the wrong kind of fats. However, partial hydrogenation not only removes essential fats, it also creates toxic fats. The problem is further exacerbated by ignorance. Most people are not aware of the health hazards that result from eating fats that have been partially hydrogenated.

History of Fats and Oils

In Europe before World War II, oil pressing was a common small business. Fresh oil was delivered from house to house once or twice a week, as were milk and eggs. In those days seed oils extracted naturally were perishable products that had to be purchased in small quantities and used within several days. Fresh oil is extremely perishable and becomes rancid very quickly.

When big business became involved, scientists discovered methods to produce oil in large volumes and to extend shelf life. The oil industry developed huge presses that generate tremendous pressure and high temperatures in the process of extracting oil from seeds.

Processing

The seed is a wonder of nature. It contains all the nutrients necessary to create new life. It is perfectly balanced. Let us see what happens when we take this nutritious seed to the oil refinery.

To begin with, the seeds are mechanically cleaned and

crushed at high temperatures. This cooking process destroys the cell walls, which makes it easier to extract the oil. The crushed, cooked seeds are then put into a huge auger press that is much like a giant kitchen meat grinder. Pressure of several tons per square inch is generated, along with temperatures of approximately 200 degrees F.

Seed oils degrade very quickly when they are exposed to heat, light, and oxygen. The large industrial processors are usually not concerned with these factors. The temperature and pressure generated in this first step of the refining process are sufficient to damage some of the sensitive fatty acids in the oil. Conditions like this produce toxic fat by-products. Before they go through any more steps in the refining process, these oils are bottled and labeled as cold-pressed, unrefined, natural oils commonly sold in health food stores. Although these oils are the best we have available, they are still adulterated.

An alternate method of removing the oil is called solvent extraction. In this process the cooked seed meal is heated under constant agitation with a solvent such as hexane, which is toxic. At the end of the process the oil is heated to about 300 degrees F to evaporate the solvent.

In the next step, the oil is degummed, which removes lecithin, chlorophyll, calcium, magnesium, iron, and copper. Then the oil is refined with a caustic corrosive chemical called sodium hydroxide (better known as a component of Drano) that helps remove the essential fatty acids.

Bleaching is the next step, providing the consumer with the colorless oil to which we are accustomed. This step also removes beta-carotene, chlorophyll, and the final traces of fatty acids. Then the oil is deodorized, which removes the distasteful odors of all the chemicals previously used. This also serves to remove the natural antioxidant, vitamin E, so critical to the oils. To counteract this loss, synthetic chemical antioxidants or preservatives such as BHA or BHT are added.

Another method used to further preserve shelf life is the process of partial hydrogenation.[3]

Partial Hydrogenation: A Major Health Hazard

The toxic fats in partially-hydrogenated fats and oils represent one of the most serious health hazards of our time because of the detrimental effects they have on our brains and bodies. The partial hydrogenation of fats and oils is an industrial process that most people do not understand. Most people are unaware of the extent that the toxic fats produced by partial hydrogenation have been introduced into our food supply. I cannot express strongly enough how important it is to read and understand this section.

To continue, the steps in the refining process thus far have removed all of nature's accessory nutrients and health-promoting substances such as minerals, lecithin, vitamin E, beta-carotene, and fiber. What is left is an isolated mixture of oils. Included in this mixture are some fats that are easily oxidized. When these oils start to become rancid, their free radical reactions will destroy the product quickly.

To decrease the likelihood of this happening and to make liquid oils more solid, the oil industry partially hydrogenates the oils. This process uses hydrogen gas under conditions of high temperature and pressure in the presence of metal catalysts. Hydrogen is forced into the structure of the fats, which actually alters the molecular structure of the fatty acids.

During the process of partial hydrogenation, the unsaturated fatty acids that do not get completely hydrogenated or saturated are twisted on a molecular level. These twisted fats have a different shape that changes their electrical and chemical properties. These toxic fats are referred to as "trans fats." Trans fats can be very dangerous to your brain and body and they should be avoided at all costs.

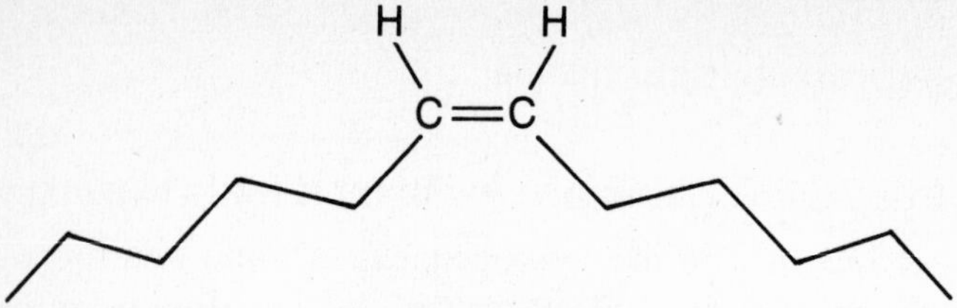

Cis-Configuration
Bent Molecule

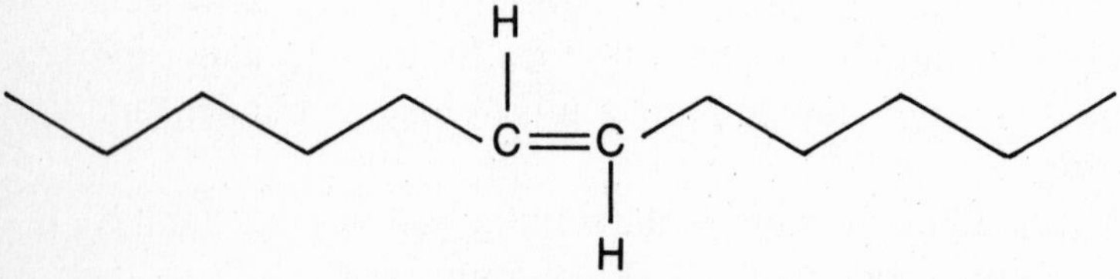

Trans-Configuration
Straight Molecule

FIGURE 12. CIS- and Trans- Configurations of Fatty Acids

CIS- and Trans- Fatty Acids

It is the change in the shape of the molecule that makes trans fats toxic. If this is the kind of fat you give to your body and brain, this is the type of fat from which your cell walls will be made. However, enzymes that take nutrients in and out of cells cannot interact with this type of fat structure. This results in improperly nourished cells causing toxic buildup within the cells.

The most commonly used partially hydrogenated products include margarine, vegetable shortenings, and shortening oils. It is estimated that margarine accounts for about 3.5 grams of partially hydrogenated fats per day in our diets and shortening accounts for another 4.6 grams. Even if you do not use margarines and shortening in your kitchen, you would be amazed by the amount of hydrogenated fats in other products you buy. Check the labels on cookies, crackers, breads, baked goods, chips, popcorn, frozen prepared foods, peanut butter, mixes for baked goods, and salad dressings. You will need to start shopping at a good, comprehensive health food store in order to avoid products containing hydrogenated fats.

Understanding Fats

Recall that we said early in this chapter that our brain cells are comprised of 60 percent fat. In a healthy, well-functioning brain, the most prevalent fats are the essential fatty acids. These fats are critical to the correct formation and maintenance of strong, flexible, semipermeable membranes of the most metabolically active brain cells. Without the correct type of fats, our brains become sluggish in their functions, memory deteriorates, and the entire body ages.

How do we get the right types of fats? How do we know which types we are ingesting? How do we avoid the potentially toxic effects of commercial fats and oils previously described? By way of answering these critical questions, allow me to give you a simple chemistry lesson on the different types of fats. Please don't become chemistry-phobic. When you understand the "why" of health issues such as these, you can make intelligent decisions in favor of health. It will longer be just a matter of self-control not to eat the "wrong" foods. It will become a personal preference.

Classification of Fats

There are a couple of different ways to classify fats. This creates some confusion that I would like to try to clear up. Fats can be classified or referred to in terms of their degree of saturation, or in terms of their essential/nonessential nature.

In terms of saturation, fats can be either saturated or unsaturated. Unsaturated fats can be further defined as monounsaturated or polyunsaturated fats. The degree of saturation refers to the number of hydrogen atoms attached to the carbon atoms in the fat molecule. When each carbon atom in the chain is linked to a hydrogen atom, we say that it is "saturated," with hydrogen atoms. When two adjacent carbon atoms on the chain do not have hydrogen atoms attached to them and instead have a "double bond" linking them, we say that it is "unsaturated."

Polyunsaturated Fatty Acid

The other method of classification refers to whether or not a particular type of fat is essential or nonessential to the biochemistry of the body. We should begin to shift away from identifying fats by degree of saturation and begin to think of fats as essential or nonessential. We do need to understand the fat-saturation concept, but it should not be the only way of determining if a fat is good for us.

The double bond is actually two pairs of electrons. At the double bond point, there is a blend in the molecule. In the cellular membranes it is this double bond and the bend in the molecule that gives the membrane its fluid, semipermeable properties. This is key to the correct functioning of brain cells and ultimately to the optimal functioning of your brain.

The double bonds are very sensitive to light, oxygen, and high temperature, and are thus easily damaged. They also are little store houses for light and energy. Hence, if you ingest more Omega-3 oils, which are highly unsaturated, you are more likely to have a higher metabolic rate and more energy. However, at the same time you risk ingesting oils that are easily oxidized, produce free radicals, and accelerate aging. This is why use of antioxidants is critical to a diet high in essential fatty acids.

Polyunsaturated oils, such as safflower, soy, and sunflower,

OMEGA-3 = ALPHA-LINOLENIC ACID

OMEGA-6 = GAMMA-LINOLENIC ACID

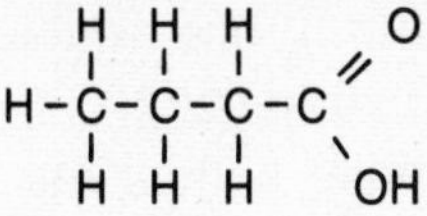

Butyric acid (butter)
A short chain saturated fatty acid

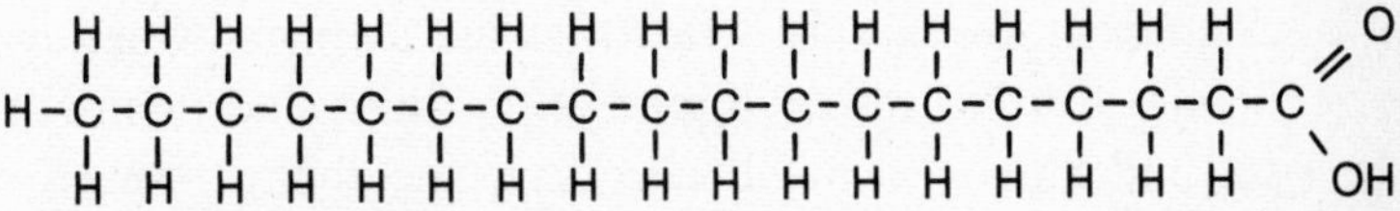

Stearic acid (large amounts in animal fats)
A long chain saturated fatty acid

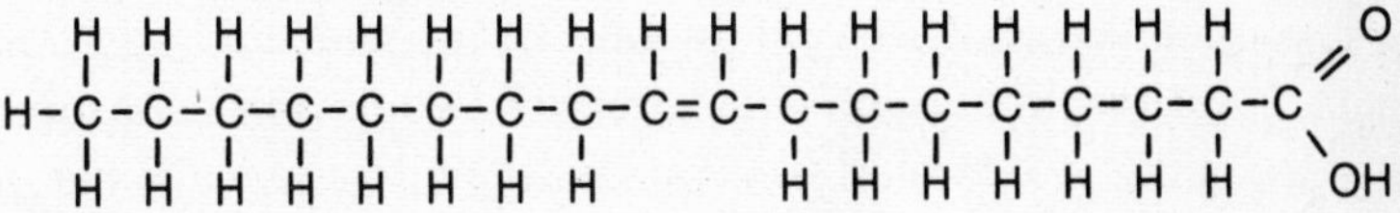

Oleic acid
A Monosaturated fatty acid (one double bond)

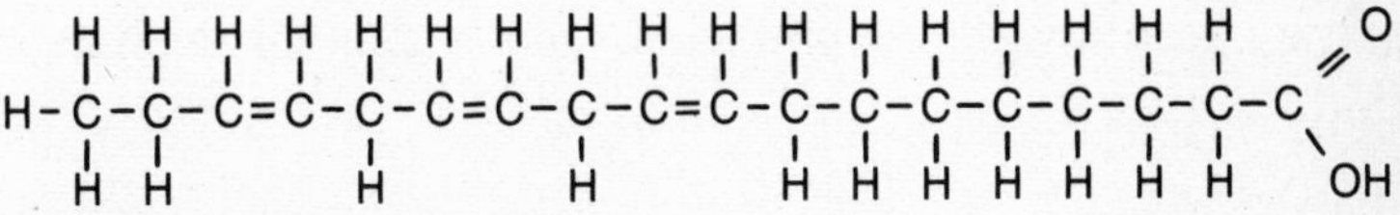

Omega-3 or alpha-linolenic acid
A polyunsaturated fatty acid (containing three double bonds)

FIGURE 13.
Structure of Saturated, Monounsaturated,
and Polyunsaturated Fatty Acids

have two or more double bonds in each fatty acid chain. Monounsaturated oils, such as olive, peanut, sesame, high oleic safflower, and high oleic sunflower, contain only one double bond, making them more stable and less easily oxidized.

Saturated fatty acids, such as butter and other animal fats, contain no double bonds. Although they are high in cholesterol, they are relatively stable. Saturated fats are nonessential fats. The body does need some saturated fats, but it can make them from the essential fatty acids. Our brains and bodies do not need the high quantity of saturated fats that the average American diet contains. Current research reports that saturated fats compete with and slow down the necessary metabolic processes involving the essential fatty acids.

Because saturated fatty acid molecules are straight chains, they pack together tightly to produce their solid, lard-like consistency. They also are lard-like in your body, which is why they do not dissolve in your blood stream and tend to form deposits on the linings of your arteries. People who consume large amounts of saturated fats essentially build cell walls out of lard. Cell walls built of hard, sticky lard-like fats do not allow for the proper passage of nutrients and toxins in and out of cells. Over time, these cells become chronically undernourished, and cannot detoxify, which results in sluggish thinking, loss of memory, cardiovascular problems, and a general decline in health.

Guidelines

Although there is a great deal of controversy surrounding the types and amounts of fats needed for optimum health, there are some simple guidelines to follow.

1. Assess your essential fatty acid intake. Most people get too much Omega-6 fats and are seriously deficient in Omega-3 fats. Supplement Omega-3 as necessary.
2. Reduce overall fat intake, especially saturated fat.

3. *Totally* avoid partially hydrogenated fats.
4. Never deep-fry or use cooking oils twice.
5. Use butter when sautéing. Olive oil, canola oil, high oleic sunflower oil, and high oleic safflower oil are acceptable for quick frying.
6. Use butter or any monounsaturated oil in baking.
7. For salads, small amounts of unfiltered, expeller-pressed vegetable oils are ideal.[4]

The important thing to realize is that the two essential fatty acids, Omega-3 (alpha-linolenic acid or Alena) and Omega-6 (linoleic acid) are the *only* two fats the body ever needs. Our bodies can make any other fat needed from these two essential fatty acids. The other thing to keep in mind is that the nonessential fatty acids are actually detrimental to your body. They interfere with, block, or inhibit the necessary metabolic processes involving the essential fatty acids.

Function of Essential Fatty Acids

The essential fatty acids perform a number of critical biological functions in the body. Let us examine how they function and why they are so important.

1. The essential fatty acids (especially Omega-3) are required for normal development of the brain and nervous system. In adults they are required for normal brain function. The human brain is about 60 percent fat. In the healthy brain Omega-3 is the most abundant fatty acid. In brain cells these semifluid fatty acids with the extra electron energy in their double bonds provide the fluidity and energy needed for proper reception and transmission of impulses between brain cells.

In the human fetus, the development of the brain and nervous system begins in the first trimester of pregnancy and is completed about one year after birth. Animal studies have shown that, when a mother's diet is deficient in Omega-3 fatty acids, her offspring show permanent learning disabilities.

Human breast milk is naturally high in Omega-3 if the mother is getting adequate Omega-3 in her diet. In comparison, cow's milk has almost no Omega-3. Furthermore, infant formulas do not contain Omega-3 fatty acids. It is very important for mothers to breast-feed their babies and to ensure that they are getting enough Omega-3 for themselves and their baby. Babies who are not breast-fed have weaker nervous systems and weaker immune systems.

In adults, Omega-3s are required for visual functioning in the retina of the eye, in synapses of the brain, in nerve tissues, in the adrenals for regulating stress, and in the testes for sperm formation.

2. These fatty acids are required for the metabolism and transport of cholesterol and triglycerides in the blood.

3. Omega-3 and Omega-6 stimulate metabolism, increase metabolic rate, increase the integration of oxygen in the cells, and increase overall energy production.

4. The essential fatty acids and their derivatives are required in the structure of cellular membranes.

5. The body uses essential fatty acids to make a group of important body chemicals called the prostaglandins.[5]

The Prostaglandins

The prostaglandins are a powerful group of hormone-like chemicals that regulate many bodily functions and activities. The prostaglandins were first discovered in the prostate gland, hence the origin of the name prostaglandins. There are now over thirty different prostaglandins that have been discovered and they are present in every organ in the body.

In his book *The Omega-3 Phenomenon*, Dr. Donald Rudin explains, "Prostaglandins are just EFAs [essential fatty acids] with a knot in their carbon chains. When EFAs are added to the deficient modern human diet, the skin, heart, kidney, liver, and reproductive organs function better. Immunity to cancer and the ability to fight infections are improved. This is because the immune system and healing are in part regulated by the action of the prostaglandins made from EFA."

The following list contains some of the activities and functions that are regulated by the prostaglandins. They:

    cause pain and stop pain.
    regulate pressure in the eye, joints, and blood vessels.
    induce labor and abortion.
    are involved with creating and relieving menstrual
        cramps.
    regulate the quantity and thickness of body secretions.
    dilate or constrict blood vessels.
    regulate smooth muscle function (such as gastrointesti-
        nal, arterial, eye, ear, and heart).
    control the blood clotting mechanism.
    regulate fever.
    affect tissue swelling.
    regulate gastric secretions and peptic ulcers.
    affect allergies and rheumatoid arthritis.
    regulate nerve transmission.
    trigger cellular division.
    control water evaporation from the skin.[6]

In order for the prostaglandins to regulate these activities at their healthiest level, Omega-3 and Omega-6 must be in proper balance. How much of each do we need to achieve this balance? According to Udo Erasmus, author of *Fats and Oils*, the optimal level of daily Omega-6 intake should be 3–5 percent of daily caloric intake. Omega-3 intake should be about 2–4 percent.

The healthy brain contains Omega-6 and Omega-3 fats in about equal amounts, or a 1:1 ratio. Estimates are that the average American diet contains about 8.5 percent Omega-6 and only about 0.4 percent Omega-3. This is a 20:1 ratio, not a 1:1 ratio. Not only is the average American diet seriously deficient

in Omega-3s, but the ratio that is so critical for proper
regulatory function is seriously out of balance.[7]

Sources and Requirements

Now that we know what the essential fatty acids are and why
they are so important, the next obvious question is where do we
get them?

The following oils are the best in descending order, nutritional sources of Omega-3 essential fatty acids: flax, pumpkin,
wheat germ, canola, soybean, and walnut. These are the only
oils that contain significant amounts of both Omega-3 and
Omega-6. Types of fish containing Omega-3 fatty acids are:
salmon, mackerel, trout, sardines, tuna, and eel.

There are a number of oils high in Omega-6 fatty acids. The
problem with these oils is that they contain virtually no
Omega-3 fatty acid, hence they promote the imbalance of the
ratio between Omega-3 and Omega-6. Oils high in Omega-6, in
descending order, are: safflower, sunflower, corn, sesame,
peanut, avocado, and olive.

Flaxseed Oil

In response to the growing awareness of the deficiency of
Omega-3 in our diets, a good-quality Omega-3 essential fatty
acid supplement is now being produced. As previously mentioned, alpha-linolenic acid is very easily destroyed by heat,
light, and exposure to oxygen. This means that a number of
special requirements have to be met in order to produce a
healthy, high quality Omega-3 product. First, special equipment that excludes light and oxygen and does not generate heat
is needed for the process. Starting with organically-grown flax,
this process produces a cold-pressed, unrefined flaxseed oil that
is light yellow in color and has a slight nutty flavor.

The product needs to be packaged in a black plastic bottle to
exclude light. Brown glass bottles are not good enough since

Essential Fatty Acid Composition
of Food Oils

Oil	Omega-3 Percentage	Omega-6 Percentage
Linseed oil	60	20
Salmon	30	20
Walnut	10	40
Wheat germ	10	40
Soybean	8	50
Safflower	1	58–75
Sunflower	1	20–72
Corn	1	40–57
Almond	1	14–44
Sesame	1	40
Avocado	1	10–40
Peanut	1	20–30
Apricot kernel	1	14–30
Olive	1	8–15
Coconut	1	2–3
Palm kernel	1	1–2

FIGURE 14.

some compounds in the oil are sensitive to longer wave lengths of light that can pass through brown glass. The bottle should also be stamped with both a pressing date and a four-month expiration date. Flaxseed oil supplements need to be refrigerated at all times.

Some companies are producing flaxseed (or linseed) oil supplements that are not of high quality. A clear or colorless oil has probably been deodorized and bleached.

Dosage

The usual recommended dosage for flaxseed oil is one table-spoonful twice daily. Some individuals with serious degenerative health problems may require more, but they should increase their dosage only with the supervision of a qualified health professional.

Fish Oils

Fish, often called brain food, is an excellent source of EPA (eicosapentanoic acid) and DHA (docosahexanoic acid), which are members of the Omega-3 fatty acid family. As we have mentioned earlier, Omega-3 plays a vital role in the healthy development and functioning of the brain and nervous system. EPA and DPA are found in high concentrations in cold-water fish, such as salmon, mackerel, sardines, tuna, and rainbow trout.[8]

Although fish oil supplements have their place, I recommend that you provide your body with oil and foods rich in linolenic acid rather than relying on fish oil supplements. I have several reasons for making this recommendation.

First, there is the problem of stability of the oils to consider. The fish oils have more double bonds in their structure, and therefore are more susceptible to rancidity. Alpha-linolenic acid is much more stable the EPA and DHA.

Second, fish oil supplements are roughly eight to twelve times more expensive than food and supplements containing linolenic acid. Due to the sensitivity of the fish oils, the costs for processing, refining, and packaging are much higher.

Third, EPA and DHA are actually derivatives of alpha-linolenic acid. It may be better to allow the body to make the conversions from alpha-linolenic acid to EPA and DHA as needed, rather than supplying it with a random amount.

There are some exceptions to this recommendation. Some people may have conditions that inhibit the conversion of linolenic acid to EPA and DHA. However, this is a genetic defect that usually occurs only in some ethnic minorities (West Coast Indians and some Japanese).

High levels of saturated fats, cholesterol, or trans-fatty acids in the diet will inhibit the conversion of Omega-3 to EPA and DHA. Elderly people, diabetics, and people with certain nutritional deficiencies such as zinc may have a greater problem with the conversion.[9] Individuals with these conditions may want to consider taking fish oil supplements.

Evening Primrose Oil

The oil of evening primrose contains a concentration of about 9 percent GLA (gamma-linolenic acid). GLA is a derivative of linoleic acid (Omega-6) and is the essential building block that the body uses in manufacturing two different groups of prostaglandins.

In some individuals, evening primrose oil can be helpful in lowering blood cholesterol and high blood pressure and in easing such conditions as arthritis, premenstrual pain, eczema, and other skin problems.[10]

Evening primrose oil can be a helpful nutritional supplement, but should not be used in place of a healthy diet that provides ample Omega-6 (linoleic acid). For people who cannot convert linoleic acid to GLA well, Evening Primrose oil as a source of GLA can be an important nutritional supplement.[11]

Caution

I need to stress the importance of understanding the potential beneficial and harmful aspects of essential fatty acids in the diet. We have discussed at length the fact that the essential Omega-3 and Omega-6 fatty acids are the only fats your body really needs. However, we have reviewed the relative instability of unsaturated fats. Thus we find ourselves in the position of needing the types of fats that are the most easily oxidized. When there is inadequate antioxidant protection in our bodies, unsaturated fats will oxidize more readily. This is at the root of the development of chronic degenerative disease and the aging process.

About forty years ago food scientists turned society in the wrong direction on this topic. When they discovered that unsaturated fats were the most easily oxidized and the most susceptible to aging, they incorrectly assumed that the best and most logical answer was to remove them from our diets. They did not realize that in addition to being the most easily destroyed, some of the unsaturated fatty acids were absolutely essential to health.

The answer to the dilemma is not to avoid the essential fatty acids, but rather to increase your protection against having that damage occur. Making sure that you have adequate levels of the key antioxidant nutrients is the answer. I believe that optimal protection should come from a combination of healthy foods in your diet and nutritional supplements.

I strongly advise people to heed this warning when taking essential fatty acid nutritional supplements. Be sure you are also taking sufficient vitamin E, beta-carotene, vitamin C, and selenium. Without proper antioxidant protection, the health benefits derived from taking flaxseed oil could be exchanged for a greater risk to some kinds of chronic degenerative diseases.

Final Comments

Many health professionals agree that the subject of fats and oils is the new frontier in gaining a deeper understanding of health. It is now known that, from birth to old age, the structure and functioning of the human brain is dependent upon the use of proper fats. Essential fatty acids are necessary for the structure of healthy brain cells as well as optimal conduction and transmission of nerve impulses. Using this new information will make a contribution to living a long life and maintaining a bright, active, functioning mind.

28

Brain Formulas: The Biochemistry of Intelligence

Spurred by interest in products that can improve intelligence, many new nutritional products are designed to enhance and increase the functioning of the brain. These formulations are designed to promote increased memory, mental acuity, and help other cognitive capabilities while slowing and preventing brain aging.

The purpose of this chapter is to discuss: (1) the ingredients in these brain/mind vitamin formulas; (2) the theory or rationale for the inclusion of these ingredients and how they function in the brain.

We will discuss the chemical compounds and reactions involved with memory and thought transmission, memory storage and retrieval, mental energy, and mental acuity. This discussion could be called the biochemistry of intelligence and memory or the biochemistry of mental functioning. To take it one step further, this is a discussion of diet and nutrition as they relate to mental functioning.

The brain is the most sensitive organ in your body. The biochemistry of intelligence depends on and is very sensitive to what you eat. Your moods and even your memory can change dramatically in response to what is eaten in a single meal. The chemical substances involved in thought processes, learning and memory processes, and other aspects of mental performance come either from your diet or are made from nutrients in the diet.

Discoveries about the relationship between nutrition and mental functioning are responsible for the recent appearance of many nutritional supplements that have been specifically designed to enhance and support the brain and mental functioning. You will recognize them when you see them. They have names like The Brain Formula, MemorAid, NutriMental, MA Formula, Brain Power, Cognitex, I.Q. Plus, and so on.

In reviewing this new class of nutritional supplements we will examine neurotransmitters, amino acids, vitamins, and a number of other substances that are used to enhance and support the brain and mental functioning and that also help to prevent brain aging.

Neurotransmitters

Neurotransmitters are chemical messengers that transmit messages between nerve cells. Neurotransmitters control a wide range of functions. In addition to thoughts and memories, they control moods such as anger, depression, and happiness. They also affect appetite, sex, sleep, and rate of breathing. However, each neurotransmitter is quite specific in its job and functions. At the beginning of the 1980s, scientists had only discovered a few neurotransmitters. Now they have found over fifty!

However, in this chapter we will focus on the neurotransmitters that are involved with memory and mental functioning.

Acetylcholine. Acetylcholine is the primary neurotransmitter involved with thought and memory. It is the chemical messenger that certain brain cells use to communicate with each other. Choline is the basis for the formation of acetylcholine. A lack of dietary choline will produce a corresponding decrease in memory. Nutritional supplementation of choline or phosphatidyl choline (lecithin) can help to restore the deficit (see Chapter 7).

Norepinephrine. Norepinephrine (NE) is another neurotransmitter that plays an important role in mental functioning. It seems to be specifically involved with long-term memory. A decrease in norepinephrine also produces a corresponding decrease in mental acuity or mental sharpness.

Two amino acids, phenylalanine and tyrosine, are used by the brain to manufacture the neurotransmitter norepinephrine. Phenylalanine is converted into tyrosine, and a second reaction converts tyrosine to norepinephrine. These two amino acids are added to many of the brain nutritional formulations. If an individual's diet is not providing enough of these two nutrient precursors, or if the supply of NE is depleted for some other reason, these amino acids will stimulate the brain to make NE.

Low levels of norepinephrine also produce depression. At one time or another we have seen someone who was depressed. Did you notice that their level of mental performance and mental sharpness were also down? People are not and cannot be in top mental form when they are depressed. The low level of norepinephrine associated with depression will produce a decrease in some areas of memory and mental functioning also.

Amino Acids

L-phenylalanine and L-tyrosine. These two amino acids have been discussed above in the section on norepinephrine (NE). Both vitamin C and vitamin B-6 are required for the conversion of these amino acids to NE. Thus, in the case of the neurotransmitter norepinephrine, we have two amino acids and two vitamins that can function therapeutically. They can be effective in enhancing memory and mental acuity, and they are also effective at relieving some types of mental depression.

Note: Individuals who may be taking medications called MAO (monoamine oxidase) inhibitors for depression should *not* use either phenylalanine or tyrosine. MAO antidepressants in combination with either phenylalanine or tyrosine can cause a dangerous elevation of blood pressure.

L-cysteine. Cysteine is a sulfur-containing, antioxidant amino acid. It is especially good at protecting the sensitive cellular membranes of the brain from free radical damage. It also protects the brain from damage due to alcohol and cigarette smoke and is a general stimulant to the immune system.

Note: The letter L in front of the names of amino acids indicates the natural form as found in nature rather than being synthetic. The L forms are more biologically active.

L-methionine. Methionine is another sulfur-containing, antioxidant amino acid that protects brain cells from damage. Methionine also prevents toxic heavy metals such as mercury and cadmium from accumulating in and damaging the brain. It plays an essential role in the production of neurotransmitters and energy production.

L-glutamine. Glutamic acid is the brain's backup or emergency source of energy. Glucose is the brain's primary source of energy. Whenever glucose is in short supply, the brain utilizes glutamic acid to keep things going. However, glutamine is the ingredient added to the brain/mind formulas, not glutamic acid. Glutamine is much more effective at getting across the blood-brain barrier than glutamic acid. Once in the brain, glutamine is converted into glutamic acid.

L-glutamine has also been effective in increasing the I.Q.s of mentally deficient children. L-glutamine is also the precursor for the neurotransmitter GABA (gamma-aminobutyric acid).

Now that we have discussed the importance of neurotransmitters and amino acids in the biochemistry of intelligence, I would like to list some of the other substances that are being used in the brain/mind nutritional formulas

Common Nutrients in Brain Formulas

Ginkgo Biloba. Its herbal extract stimulates cerebral circulation and improves mental functioning (see Chapter 17).

RNA (Ribonucleic Acid). The synthesis of RNA is required for memory. Animal studies suggest that RNA supplements may improve memory.

Vitamin B-1 (Thiamine). Thiamine is essential for the health of brain and nerve tissue. It is also involved in the chemical reactions that cause the release of acetylcholine in the brain.

Vitamin B-2 (Riboflavin). Riboflavin functions as an antioxidant cofactor, taking part in the antioxidant reactions involving both superoxide dismutase (SOD) and glutathione peroxidase.

Vitamin B-3 (Niacin). A deficiency of niacin produces memory failure. It functions in over fifty metabolic reactions, especially those producing energy. Niacin has two forms, nicotinic acid and niacinamide. Either or both forms can be utilized in nutritional formulations.

Vitamin B-5 (Pantothenic Acid). Vitamin B-5 acts as an antioxidant. It is also required for the conversion of choline to acetylcholine.

Vitamin B-6 (Pyridoxine). Vitamin B-6 acts as an antioxidant. It is also required for the conversion of amino acids into neurotransmitters in the brain. For example, the conversion of phenylalanine to norepinephrine requires vitamin B-6.

Vitamin B-12 (Cobalamin). Vitamin B-12 is a coenzyme that is particularly important in the brain and nerve tissues. It is necessary for the synthesis of DNA and RNA; it enhances the action of vitamin C and several amino acids; and it is required to build the walls of brain cells.

Vitamin C (Ascorbic Acid). Vitamin C is a major antioxidant. It is a precursor for the production of the neurotransmitters norepinephrine, epinephrine, and serotonin. For example, the production of norepinephrine has been shown to be severely inhibited in vitamin C-deficient subjects (see Chapter 21).

Vitamin E. Vitamin E is a powerful lipid membrane antioxidant that protects brain cells from free radical damage (see Chapter 23).

Folic acid. Folic acid is selectively concentrated in the brain and spinal fluid and is essential to the functioning of the brain. It functions as a coenzyme in the production of norepinephrine, and is necessary for the synthesis of DNA and RNA. It is also essential for the synthesis of methionine in the brain.

Biotin. Biotin acts as a coenzyme in many reactions and also helps to fight mild depression.

Inositol. Inositol is a membrane stabilizer found in high concentrations in the cellular tissue of the brain. It reportedly promotes an anti-anxiety or calming effect.

L-phenylalanine. Phenylalanine is a precursor for the neurotransmitter norepinephrine.

L-tyrosine. Tyrosine is a precursor for the neurotransmitter norepinephrine.

L-methionine. Methionine is an antioxidant sulfur-containing amino acid.

L-cysteine. Cysteine is an antioxidant sulfur-containing amino acid.

DMAE (Dimethylaminoethanol). DMAE enhances memory and intelligence. It is a source of choline for the production of acetylcholine in the brain (see Chapter 8).

Germanium. Germanium is an important nutritional discovery that appears to aid in the oxygenation of cells and tissue.

Phosphatidlyserine. Evidence indicates that phosphatidlyserine helps improve memory and prevent age-related memory loss. It actually resides in brain cell membranes where it activates the release of acetylcholine and enhances the transmission of nerve messages between brain cells.

Potassium. Potassium is responsible for transmitting electrical impulses. It is highly active in the tissues of the brain and nervous system.

Zinc. The brain contains substantial concentrations of zinc. It is a necessary cofactor in over twenty different enzymatic reactions and is essential for the production of the antioxidant enzyme SOD. It also helps prevent the accumulation of lead that is toxic to the brain.

Manganese. Manganese is a cofactor in many enzyme mediated reactions. It is essential for the production of the antioxidant enzyme SOD (see Chapter 4).

Octacosanol. Octacosanol has been shown to improve the body's ability to utilize oxygen, to improve reaction time, and improve performance under stress.

Chromium. Chromium is essential for the metabolism of glucose and the production of energy.

Taurine. Taurine is a nonessential amino acid possessing a bipolar chemical structure. Its bipolar nature reportedly enables it to function as a charge stabilizer in the conduction of electrical impulses along nerve pathways.

Final Comments

This chapter was designed as a reference to help individuals evaluate and understand the ingredients in this new class of nutritional supplements.

Proper functioning of the neurotransmitters is the key to optimal memory, mental acuity, and mental functioning. The amino acids, vitamins, and other accessory nutrients provide the necessary foundation to support optimal functioning of the brain.

Some products are formulated to enhance memory, some are formulated for mental acuity, and others are designed to increase mental energy. These products represent a growing awareness of the need to provide good nutritional support for our minds as well as our bodies.

The Aging Brain: Senility and Alzheimer's Disease

As the brain ages, it definitely changes. However, the results of these changes are not always devastating. There are a number of misconceptions about the aging brain and elderly people. In this chapter I will describe the brain changes that occur with aging. Then I will discuss some myths and misconceptions about the aging process and the aging brain. Next we will examine the conditions called senility and dementia. Finally, we will discuss the special case of senility called Alzheimer's disease.

Changes in the Aging Brain

There are a number of fairly predictable changes in the aging brain. With age, the brain becomes physically smaller and lighter. This decrease in size and weight actually causes the brain to become looser in the skull cavity. Could this be where the expression "rattle your brain" comes from?

In a normal lifetime, billions of brain cells, or neurons will die. Dr. Arnold Scheibel at the Department of Anatomy at UCLA is a pioneer in brain research. He has shown that from 20 to 40 percent of the cells in areas of the brain involved with memory can be lost by the age of ninety. Of even greater significance, he found that many of the brain cells had lost up

ANTIAGING

to 80 percent of their fine network of branch-like extensions called neurites or dendrites. These are the structures that communicate with neighboring brain cells.[1]

Cellular garbage deposits called lipofuscin or "age pigment" continue to accumulate in brain cells throughout life. The exact nature and effect they have on cellular function is not totally understood, but it is clear that lipofuscin deposits are definitely a sign of aging.

Sometimes groups of cells in the aging brain can degenerate into masses called neuritic plaques. Nerves and nerve fibers get twisted into clusters called neurofibrillary tangles.

There is also a large reduction in neurotransmitters in the aging brain. The brain in healthy aged individuals has been shown to have up to 70 percent decrease in acetylcholine.

Healthy Aging vs. Unhealthy Aging: The Good News

Yes, there is good news to report. The physical changes in the aging brain do not occur at the same rate or to the same degree in everyone. Even better news is that the changes discussed above do not always lead to a predictable decline and deterioration in the behavior and functional capacity of the individual.

This leads us into a discussion of some of the myths and misconceptions about aging and senility. A study titled *Human Aging* was conducted by the National Institute of Mental Health (NIMH). The results from this study have disproved some common beliefs about aging and its relationship to mental health and intellectual performance.

The volunteers for this study were elderly men (average age seventy-one) and extremely healthy for their age. Two weeks of extensive medical examinations were conducted before starting the study. Results of the medical exams revealed that twenty of the original forty-seven volunteers had some minor health problems. The members of this subgroup had no symptoms, felt fine, and were unaware of any health problems. These two groups of men were then followed from 1957 to 1968. I will refer to these two groups as the totally healthy group and the almost totally healthy group.

After eleven years of tracking, the researchers found a significant decline in the brain function in the almost totally healthy group. However, results from the totally healthy group of men (many who were now in their eighties) astounded the investigators. These men scored about the same in brain function as normal, healthy young adults![2]

The results from the *Human Aging* study have struck a blow at some of the long-held stereotypes about old age. The *Human Aging* study discovered that senility is not a necessary part of aging, but that it is associated with the physical degeneration that frequently accompanies old age. In other words, elderly people who are healthy do not lose their minds or their memories. In fact, noted gerontologist Alex Comfort stated that elderly humans who remain healthy can look forward to normal sexual functioning and normal intelligence throughout their entire lifetime.[3]

In addition to the physical and structural changes already mentioned, there are two changes that occur in the aging brain that do produce a functional decline in the aging individual. There is a gradual decline in both memory and the speed of response. However, in normal aging, the decline in these functions is usually mild. Individuals should be counseled and cautioned to expect this slight decline without expecting it to progress into a crippling problem.

Benign Forgetfulness

Psychologists now divide memory loss into two categories. There is benign memory loss and malignant memory loss. Benign forgetfulness occurs when you forget where you left your car keys; malignant forgetfulness occurs when you forget that you own a car. The point here is that benign forgetfulness should be expected and understood. Many elderly individuals project themselves into needless fear over normal episodes of benign forgetfulness.

Benign forgetfulness can be compensated for by recognizing the need to develop helpful ways to aid memory. Learn to post notes to help you remember and leave something you want to take with you in front of the door. When you start forgetting telephone numbers and addresses and make more frequent use of telephone books, there is no need to be ashamed of it. You can even have people call to remind you of appointments. Memory may slip with age, but in many cases, the aged person can still live and function very well.

Senility and Dementia

Senility and dementia are terms used to describe a group of symptoms and behaviors related to intellectual deterioration. In simple terms, intellectual deterioration means the loss of memory and the ability to think. There are over seventy recognized diseases and disorders that can cause these symptoms and behavioral changes.

In 1980 the American Psychiatric Association (APA) published the third edition of its *Diagnostic and Statistical Manual of Mental Disorders* (or *DSM-III*). This publication sets the criteria and standards for the diagnosis of dementia. According to the standards set by DSM-III, the diagnosis of dementia requires that an individual have an impairment in memory and an impairment in at least one other area of cognition.[4]

The diagnostic criteria for the diagnosis of dementia are:
1. A loss of intellectual abilities
2. Impaired social or occupational function
3. Memory impairment
4. Impairment of additional areas of cognition (personality change or loss of knowledge and use of language skills)
5. State of consciousness (clouded vs. alert and awake)
6. Evidence of organic damage

There is still some disagreement among professionals about the standards used to determine dementia. For example, mental tests that can be used to help confirm dementia were not used to set the DSM-III standards. Several other professional groups have developed diagnostic criteria that differ slightly from DSM-III. Even though some disagreements exist, tremendous advances have been made in the last decade in our ability to diagnose dementia correctly.

Reversible Causes of Senility

To date most of the seventy diseases that can produce the complex of symptoms called senility or dementia seem to be irreversible. However, physicians and the general public should be aware of the fact that there are a number of causes of senility that are reversible. The general categories of reversible causes of senility are psychiatric disorders, drugs, metabolic disorders, and nutritional disorders. Each will be discussed briefly.

Psychiatric Disorders

Psychiatric disorders sometimes create a form of dementia that is treatable. Depression, sensory deprivation, and other psychiatric conditions fall into this category. Depression is the most common.

A landmark study in 1974 by psychiatrist Robert Kahn shed a great deal of light on the issue of memory loss associated with aging. He administered memory tests and psychiatric tests to a group of elderly psychiatric patients and made two startling discoveries. First, he found that, in individuals with no signs of actual brain dysfunction, those who complained the most about their memory problems actually had memories that tested and functioned just fine. Second, he found that those individuals who saw themselves as most forgetful were not forgetful, they were depressed.[5]

Psychosocial and environmental conditions often produce

depression in the elderly. In our society the elderly often have to cope with difficult situations such as poor housing, lack of friends, lack of respect, low incomes, and lack of care. These problems can create depression and fear that can easily influence thinking and memory. In the elderly these behaviors are often diagnosed as senility. When understood and treated correctly, the patient often improves.

Drugs

Many classes of drugs are known to cause the symptoms of senility. There are many variables involved with these cases such as the length of time taking the drug, the strength and dosage of the drug, and the patient's individual physical condition.

It is beyond the scope of this book to list all the drugs that have been known to produce these symptoms. I will list some of the main classes of drugs to be cautious of. They are:

1. Sedatives or sleep medications
2. Antidepressants
3. Tranquilizers
4. Antiarrhythmics or heart medications
5. Antihypertensives or blood pressure medication
6. Anticonvulsants for epilepsy.[6]

Therapy for individuals who develop dementia from any of these classes of drugs usually involves discontinuing and/or changing medications. Dietary changes and nutritional supplementation usually are needed as well. If you know someone who is displaying symptoms of senility, it might be wise to check the type and quantity of medications they are taking and consult with their physician.

Metabolic Disorders

A number of metabolic disorders can create the symptoms of senility. Correct diagnosis of these conditions requires the attention of a physician and laboratory diagnostic procedures. Because of their technical nature they will only be listed here. The main metabolic disorders are:

1. Hypo- and hyperthyroidism (thyroid hormones)
2. Hypercalcemia (high calcium levels)
3. Hypo- and hypernatremia (high or low sodium)
4. Hypoglycemia (low blood sugar levels)
5. Hyperlipidemia (high fat levels)
6. Hypercapnia (carbon dioxide)
7. Kidney failure
8. Liver failure

These conditions frequently can be treated with diet, nutrition, and lifestyle changes under the supervision of a competent health professional.[7]

Nutritional Disorders

The final group of reversible causes of senility is nutritional disorders. It is well known that some nutritional deficiencies can produce symptoms of mental illness. However, it is important to note that the process of aging does not create nutritional deficiencies. Carefully controlled studies comparing young adults with the elderly (average age of seventy) who were selected for their high level of health revealed no significant differences in nutritional requirements for vitamins, minerals or the principle macronutrients.[8]

The nutritional disorders that can cause symptoms of senility are the following:

1. Pellagra (vitamin B-3 or niacin deficiency). Vitamin B-3 is found in significant amounts in meat, poultry, legumes, milk, and eggs.
2. Beriberi (vitamin B-1 or thiamine deficiency). Vitamin B-1 is found in significant amounts in pork, beef, whole wheat, nuts, peas, and beans.
3. Pernicious anemia (vitamin B-12 or cobalamin defi-

ciency). The best dietary sources of vitamin B-12 are organ meats (liver, kidney, heart), crab, salmon, sardines, and egg yolk.

4. Folic acid deficiency (a B-vitamin). Good dietary sources of folic acid are green vegetables, organ meats, cabbage, yeast, cauliflower, wheat germ, and whole-grain products.[9]

Drug-Induced Nutritional Deficiencies

The elderly are by far the largest consumers of drugs (both prescription and nonprescription) in the United States. Most of these drug-induced nutritional deficiencies will not directly produce the symptoms of senility and dementia. We do not know exactly to what degree nutritional deficiencies (major or minor) throughout life might contribute to the deterioration of mental functioning later in life. However, it is well known that nutrition is an essential factor in the rate of aging and disease, determining both the quality and the length of life.

A listing of some of the more important and/or more common potential drug-induced nutritional deficiencies follows:

1. Penicillin antibiotics can cause a deficiency in vitamins B-6, B-12, folic acid, vitamin K, and potassium.

2. Tetracycline antibiotics can cause a deficiency in vitamins B-2, B-6, B-12, folic acid, vitamin C, calcium, iron, magnesium, and zinc.

3. Erythromycin antibiotics can cause a deficiency in vitamins B-6, B-12, folic acid, vitamin K, calcium, and magnesium.

4. Many diuretics deplete potassium, zinc, magnesium, calcium, and iodine.

5. Potassium replacement for people taking diuretics causes a depletion of vitamin B-12.

6. Indocin for arthritis depletes iron.

7. Tagamet for ulcers depletes iron.

8. Dilantin for epilepsy depletes vitamins K, D, and folic acid.

9. Lanoxin for the heart depletes zinc and vitamin B-1.

10. Aluminum antacids such as Maalox, Gelusil, and Di-Gel inhibit the absorption of calcium, phosphorus, magnesium iron, and vitamins A, C, D, and B-1.

11. Calcium antacids like Tums inhibit the absorption of phosphorus, magnesium, folic acid, iron, and vitamin B-1.

12. Premarin for estrogen can cause a deficiency in vitamins B-2, B-6, B-12, C, and folic acid.

13. Many over-the-counter laxatives can inhibit the absorption of potassium, calcium, and vitamin D.

14. Aspirin irritates the lining of the stomach and can cause bleeding. A couple of aspirin can cause the loss of about 1 teaspoon of blood and 2 mg of iron.[10]

Treatment of the drug-induced nutritional deficiencies usually involves discontinuation of the drug creating the problem and using nutritional supplementation to overcome the deficiencies.

Alzheimer's Disease

Alzheimer's disease is only one of the more than seventy different disorders and diseases that can cause the symptoms of senility. However, Alzheimer's disease is by far the most significant of these disorders because it accounts for 50 to 60 percent of the known cases. The disease is sometimes referred to as senile dementia Alzheimer's type (SDAT) or dementia Alzheimer's type (DAT).

In 1906 the German physician Alois Alzheimer observed and described a set of characteristic clinical and neuropathological symptoms that now bears his name. A 1982 publication from the National Institutes of Health describes Alzheimer's disease as follows:

It develops gradually and steadily rather than suddenly. Clinical diagnosis is based on the occurrence of a sequence of characteristic symptoms. Loss of memory for recent events is usually the first sign of the disorder, followed by impairment of judgement, comprehension and other cognitive functions, which usually occurs within one year. Anxiety, depression and other emotional disturbances often follow. Intellectual deterioration slowly worsens, and symptoms of neurological impairment, such as difficulty in walking begin to appear. Finally, the patient becomes bedridden with a deep dementia. Death usually occurs from infection or some other complication about 5 to 8 years after the onset of the disease.[11]

The electron microscope now enables scientists to see structural changes in brain cells. The brains of individuals who have died from Alzheimer's disease contain structural changes called neuritic plaques and neurofibrillary tangles. Neuritic plaques consist of a central core of protein material surrounded by degenerated cellular fragments. The neurofibrillary tangles are bundles of nerve filaments from brain cells that twist and wind around each other. Together these micropathologic changes are referred to as "Alzheimer-type brain changes."[12]

Another characteristic change in the brains of individuals with Alzheimer's disease is the accumulation of aluminum. Scientists have not been able to prove that the accumulation of brain aluminum levels causes Alzheimer's disease. All we can say is that there is an association between the accumulation of aluminum in the brain and Alzheimer's disease.

Alzheimer's Disease: Cause and Treatment

The cause of Alzheimer's disease remains a mystery. We can examine the degenerative changes in the brain structure, we can measure the decrease in neurotransmitters, we know the aluminum is there, and we can observe the functional and behavioral changes in the patients. But the cause is still a mystery.

Some researchers have suggested that latent viruses could be a possible cause. The fact that about 10 percent of the cases are familial begs the question of a possible genetic link. The search for a cause and more accurate ways to diagnose Alzheimer's disease continues to be a major focus of current medical research.

Unfortunately, there is still no effective treatment for advanced cases of Alzheimer's disease. However new research suggests that some progress is being made in the understanding and treatment of this disease.

Naltrexone

Dr. Forest Tennant from the UCLA School of Public Health has recently published encouraging new work in this area. Dr. Tennant has been very successful in treating individuals with drug addictions. He "stumbled" onto the fact that some drugs that function as narcotic antagonists provided improvement of symptoms in Alzheimer's patients.

Naltrexone is a long-acting narcotic antagonist that is capable of remaining in the body for up to seventy-two hours. Dr. Tennant has conducted preliminary trials with Naltrexone, treating Alzheimer's patients for from two to six months. He used two standardized tests to assess progress, the MiniMental Test (MMT) and the Blessed Dementia Scale (BDS). Most of his subjects have improved from 10 to 50 percent within the first sixty days of treatment.[13]

The families of these Alzheimer's patients report also improvements in patient's memory, mental status, and living functions. The families often request that their family member remain on the therapy.

Dr. Tennant has administered choline to his patients along with the Naltrexone. It is not certain if choline contributes a therapeutic effect, but if Naltrexone stimulates neurons to release acetylcholine, then administration of choline may help to prevent depletion of the neurotransmitter.

Symmetrel (Amantadine)

Dr. Tennant has also been using amantadine to treat Alzheimer's disease. Amantadine, also marketed under the trade
name Symmetrel, is primarily known as an antiviral medication. Its ability to affect some neurotransmitters is presumably
a partial explanation of its mechanism of action. In a pamphlet
titled *Medical Treatment for Alzheimer's Disease*, Dr. Tennant
says, "The most successful medications in our program have
been Naltrexone and amantadine. These two drugs, particularly
in combination, have been able to improve symptoms in about
80 percent of the Alzheimer's cases. There have been no
significant side effects to date, and we have high hopes that it
may even slow the progression of Alzheimer's disease.

In a taped interview, Dr. Tennant openly urged doctors to try
all Alzheimer's patients with either one or both of these drugs
for one to three months. The cost is reasonable, there are not
many side effects and the percentage of patients responding
positively has been very high.[14]

Several therapies that have been able to produce some
improvement in cases that are diagnosed early have already
been discussed in individual chapters earlier in this book. These
are the chapters on choline/lecithin, Hydergine, Lucidril, cognitive enhancers, piracetam, and the combination of piracetam
and choline.

Alzheimer's Disease and Nutrition

Is there an answer to this medical/economic/social/emotional
dilemma called Alzheimer's disease? The cure is not in sight.
However, some new insights about the relationship between
Alzheimer's disease and the nutritional status of the patient are
coming to light. This nutritional association between the patient
and the disease may provide some important clues to the
treatment and prevention of this disease.

The Calcium/Aluminum Connection

Consider the following. We know that the brain of the patient with Alzheimer's disease frequently contains high levels of aluminum. It is known that aluminum concentrates to a higher degree in the nerve tissue of individuals who are low in calcium. The low calcium intake seems to produce an endocrine imbalance called hyperparathyroidism. This imbalance encourages the uptake of aluminum into the nervous tissue of the brain.

The accumulation of aluminum produces two other changes. First, it alters the activity of the enzyme acetylcholinesterase, reducing the amount of the neurotransmitter acetylcholine in the brain. Second, aluminum initiates free radical damage in the brain tissue.[15]

Thus, we have three conditions directly related to Alzheimer's disease (high levels of aluminum in the brain, high levels of free radical damage, and low levels of acetylcholine), which are all related to the nutritional problem of low levels of calcium.

The Vitamin B-12 Connection

A psychiatrist, Dr. Van Tigelan, discovered an important condition in his patients that were suffering from Alzheimer's disease. He found that their cerebral spinal fluid levels of vitamin B-12 were extremely low, even though they had normal vitamin B-12 levels in their blood. It was stated earlier in this chapter that cobalamin or vitamin B-12 deficiency can cause dementia. When he gave these Alzheimer's patients vitamin B-12 injections he observed both an elevation in their cerebral spinal fluid B-12 levels and clinical improvement of their symptoms. Dr. Van Tigelan suggests that these patients may have a transport problem in getting B-12 into the spinal fluid and on to the brain.[16]

This study points out that some individuals may have transport problems with certain nutrients and the clinical impact this may have in relationship to brain chemistry. It also alerts us to the fact that laboratory values from blood and urine samples may not tell us what is going on in certain organs and tissues, especially the brain.

The Vitamin C Connection

Dr. Irwin Stone is one of the leading pioneers in researching vitamin C and its important health-related benefits. It was Dr. Stone who originally introduced vitamin C to Dr. Linus Pauling. They have been close friends and colleagues ever since. The following comments are summarized from an article by Dr. Stone that was published in the May 1983 issue of *Anti-Aging News*. The title of that article is: "Ascorbic Acid Therapy for Aging and Alzheimer's Disease."

In 1959 it was discovered that almost all species of mammals contain a series of four enzymes which enables them to synthesize vitamin C in the liver. It was also discovered that the last in this series of four enzymes is missing in the human liver. The missing enzyme in humans is probably the result of an unfortunate genetic mutation that occurred millions of years ago in our evolutionary history. This change renders us unable to synthesize vitamin C.

Dr. Stone believes that the loss of the ability to make vitamin C creates a condition called hypo-ascorbemia (low vitamin C) which afflicts virtually 100 percent of the human population. In light of this, he has said, "the current RDA for vitamin C of 60 mg a day is low by a factor of over two hundred and under stress may rise to the thousands."

In his article, Dr. Stone also said, "Alzheimer's disease is just another disease on the long list of current medical problems having its origin, high morbidity, and high mortality due to chronic physiologic insults from subclinical scurvy.

"By a simple urine test it can be shown that untreated

potential and actual Alzheimer's disease victims also suffer from more or less severe cases of chronic subclinical scurvy.[17] In the many abortive attempts at treating Alzheimer's disease in the past, clinical investigators have failed to eradicate this deadly genetic syndrome, even though I described Hypoascorbemia in 1966. Since Scurvy is the most misunderstood disease in modern medicine, it is the last syndrome to come under suspicion as the cause of modern diseases.[18]

"In Alzheimer's disease, death usually occurs from infection or other complication about five to eight years after the onset of the disease. It should be remembered that lack of resistance to infections is a classic symptom of scurvy, known for centuries. The scorbutic human immune system functions at a very low level of efficiency in the production of defensive immune factors. This can be reversed with the proper daily intake of ascorbate."[19]

Final Comments

I must emphasize that, to date, the therapies for Alzheimer's disease can only help; they do not cure the disease, nor can they reverse the damage that has been done.

Even though some therapies show a glimmer of promise, the cause of Alzheimer's disease remains a mystery and treatment is generally limited to management of the symptoms. I know of no other condition where it is more important to consider the overall medical, social, economic, emotional, and spiritual needs of the patient and the family than with Alzheimer's disease. The stresses in caring for a patient with this disease are so great that the care-givers are often driven to the breaking point. This is another significant concern related to this disease.

Alzheimer's disease has been called the disease of the century.[20] The following comments are an attempt to give you some idea of the magnitude of the problem. The social, economic, and emotional dimensions of this disease are staggering. Surveys indicate that Alzheimer's disease is the major cause for institutionalization among the more than one million persons in nursing homes in the United States. A fact that makes these figures even more dramatic is that there are more patients in nursing homes than there are in *all* the hospitals in the United States. And yet, the nursing home population represents only a fraction of the problem. Thousands more are confined to state institutions and V.A. hospitals. Many more are cared for at home by relatives and friends. And finally there are the uncounted thousands who are alone and confused, often existing in terrible living conditions, and unable to find or get help.

Alzheimer's disease is primarily a disease of the elderly. Changing demographics resulting in "the graying of America" contribute to the increasing number of diagnosed cases. In 1986 approximately 2 to 2.5 million Americans were afflicted with Alzheimer's disease. The number of afflicted individuals will increase proportionately as the older segment of our population grows. The diagnosed cases of Alzheimer's disease are expected to double in the next forty years. This is an approaching epidemic.

30

Conclusion

Three relatively new and important areas of science and health have been addressed in this research:

1. Nutrients and drugs that enhance intelligence
2. The free radical theory of aging
3. Life extension and antiaging

These three areas are clearly interrelated. They are the foundation of a program to enhance mental functioning, increase intelligence, and significantly decrease both the rate at which the brain ages and the loss of intelligence with aging.

The free radical theory of aging provides an explanation of the cause of damage to cellular membranes and cellular components. There is ample evidence to suggest that this type of damage is the source of biological aging. The following summary may serve to provide a more complete understanding of the research in this work, and help to suggest and stimulate further research related to the material presented here.

Free radical reactions are a life-and-death drama that continually occurs at the cellular level. An in-depth exploration of the various types of free radicals and the chemistry of their reactivity is beyond the scope of this study. However, a basic explanation of how antioxidants can prevent uncontrollable free radical chain reactions was presented in Chapter 4.

Free radical reactions constitute an ongoing source of cellular damage in all species that utilize oxygen. It is a paradox that oxygen, which is essential for all animal life, can also be toxic. When the optimal supply of oxygen to the cells and tissues is upset, conditions are created that allow it to react with and damage membrane lipids and other cellular components such as DNA and RNA. The brain and central nervous system, which contain the highest levels of unsaturated fats, are especially susceptible to free radical damage. This means that our brains and our intelligence are the primary targets of destruction from free radical reactions.

Antioxidants can scavenge or neutralize free radicals and thus prevent the initiation of uncontrolled free radical chain reactions. An understanding of the relationship between free radicals and antioxidants enables us to exert control over our own individual level of health and our aging process.

Many chemical and physical agents in the environment can serve to initiate free radical reactions, and there are a number of different types of free radicals capable of being generated. Through optimal nutrition and a healthy life style, exposure to free radicals can be minimized and much of the damage they cause can be prevented. Understanding the importance of free radicals and antioxidants can lead to the formulation of a program promoting high level wellness, life extension in terms of both quantity and quality, and the maintenance of optimal intelligence and mental function throughout life.

Denham Harman, the originator of the free radical theory of aging, has said that aging is our number one health problem, and statistics seem to support his statement. For example, in 1966, national health costs in the United States totaled $47.1 billion—in 1984, that figure reached $360 billion. The average health expenditure for each individual was $211 in 1966. In 1981, it had risen to $1,225 per person. A more staggering statistic relates to health care costs for the elderly. In 1966 the average health care expenditure for each elderly person was $300—by 1981, it had risen to an incredible $2,395 per person.

These are sad statistics when one considers the cumulative

loss of health, happiness, intellectual capabilities, and worker productivity, as well as money. With an understanding of the free radical theory of aging, we are beginning to see that chronic degenerative diseases are preventable. This highlights a need at both the individual and the national level for a paradigm shift in our thinking about health and our programs for health education. The emphasis must shift from treating individual cases of chronic degenerative disease after they have appeared to detecting the early warning signs and paying attention to prevention through diet, exercise, and general life style modification.

The purpose of this study was to investigate the effects of certain nutrients and drugs on the enhancement of intelligence and the retardation of brain aging. A summary of important information about the drugs and nutrients discussed in this book is given in Figure 15.

This research is not meant to be "the answer" to aging or our ability to enhance intelligence. Research into the mechanisms of aging and human intelligence is just beginning. As we have just scratched the surface with some initial successes in life extension and increasing intelligence, the need for more research is obvious. It seems that the more we learn, the more we need to learn.

It is exciting to realize that intelligence is not static. The "elasticity" of the brain is now being explored. As some brain cells die, others continue to grow and increase their dendritic connections. New drugs and combinations of drugs and brain nutrients wait to be explored. If we expand Luis Machado's phrase "Intelligence is learned, not bred" to include a deeper understanding of the biochemistry of intelligence, the potential benefit to society is enormous.

Another important task this research brings to light is the fact that what is already known in isolated areas of science must be organized and communicated in an understandable way to both

Summary of the Intelligence-Enhancing and Antiaging Effects of the Nutrients, Herbs, and Drugs Discussed in This Book

Name	Classification	Available in U.S.	Treats Senility	Helps Prevent Memory Loss	Prevents Free Radical Damage	Improves Memory and Learning	Special Effects
Choline/Lecithin	N	X	X	X		X	None
DMAE	N	X	X	X		X	Mood elevation
Diapid	Rx	X				X	Increases short-term memory
Hydergine	Rx	X	X	X	X	X	Increases oxygen supply to brain tissue
Lucidril	Rx		X	X	X	X	Rejuvenates nerve synapses, removes aging deposits
Piracetam	Rx			X	X	X	Increases interhemispheric communication
Vitamin C	N	X		X	X		Major antioxidant nutrient
Vitamin E	N	X		X	X		Major antioxidant nutrient
Beta-carotene/Vitamin A	N	X		X	X		Major antioxidant nutrient
Selenium	N	X		X	X		Strong anticancer nutrient, major antioxidant nutrient
Ginseng	H	X				X	Adaptogen
Ginkgo biloba	H	X		X	X		Increases circulation to microcapillaries
Dilantin/DPH	Rx	X				X	Normalizes and stabilizes electrical energy in the brain

N = nutrient   Rx = prescription drug   H = herb

FIGURE 15.

the medical and scientific communities, as well as to the general public.

The statistics on health care costs indicate that the current approach to health care has serious flaws. The financial burden alone is forcing us to reevaluate the direction of the present health care system and what it has (or has not) been accomplishing.

A historical perspective allows us to understand how the present crisis developed. Louis Pasteur discovered that germs caused disease. In the following century antibiotics were developed that killed the germs and restored health. Based on these successes, an entire generation developed the belief that research can find and develop a specific drug that will cure any disease. The miracle cure from the doctor worked well; it conquered infectious diseases.

However, times and the problems have changed. The current situation needs to be viewed from a different perspective. Medicine can be cleanly divided into two basic areas.

1. Acute or emergency care—i.e. infectious diseases, cuts, infections, broken bones, etc.
2. The treatment of chronic degenerative disease.

Western medicine excels in the treatment of acute and emergency medicine. However, the World Health Organization (WHO) estimates that over 80 percent of the deaths in the United States are due to chronic degenerative diseases. This emphasizes the fact that Western medicine has failed in its attempts to treat chronic degenerative diseases. We are learning the hard way; old beliefs die hard. Finally we are beginning to learn that prevention, not treatment, is the cure.

The "new" approaches to health care carry names like preventive medicine, holistic health, orthomolecular medicine, and nutritional biochemistry. These approaches attempt to pinpoint early warning signs long before a disease manifests.

The use of nutrients, herbs, and drugs to increase intelligence and extend life constitutes a relatively new area of scientific research. Although research in these areas is just beginning, initial successes and the promise of future benefits have created an air of excitement among those who are involved directly.

The research reported in this book points out some general areas where more research is needed. More work is needed to determine optimal dosage levels of the drugs, herbs, and nutrients that have already shown positive results. More research into the long-term effects and the optimal length of therapy is needed. The whole area of using combinations of drugs, herbs, and nutrients to get additive synergistic effects awaits further exploration.

There is a need for more research in several specific areas:

Hydergine. Long-term effects need to be evaluated to determine how effectively it prevents the loss of intelligence with age and if its ability to minimize free radical damage will translate into life extension.

Lucidril. What is the optimal length of time it should take to remove deposits of lipofuscin? Is the optimal length of administration related to the amount of lipofuscin accumulated? Should it be taken periodically or continually to prevent lipofuscin buildup? The p-chlorophenoxy-acetate part of the centrophenoxine molecule needs to be evaluated to determine what part it plays in producing the benefits obtained through its use.

Piracetam. Its long-term effects need to be evaluated for both intelligence enhancement and antiaging benefits. The significance of piracetam's ability to superconnect the brain by facilitating the transfer of information between the left and right hemispheres of the brain needs to be explored. This raises the question of whether superconnecting the cerebral hemispheres can increase insightfulness and creativity.

New Drugs. Research is needed to develop new drugs with potential for enhancing intelligence and mental functioning and to explore the use of new synergistic combinations.

I hope this book will increase public awareness for the need for a shift in national policy regarding the funding of research in these areas. Currently, approximately 95 percent of the government funds for health research is awarded to support research into the development of new drugs to treat specific diseases or into new technology for such things as artificial hearts and organ transplants. The cancer industry alone spends billions of dollars on research. Unfortunately, less than 5 percent of the available funds are awarded to support research in the area of prevention and wellness. Almost nothing goes to intelligence enhancement or life extension.

For centuries the possibilities of increasing intelligence and extending life have been regarded as mere fantasy. Now, for the first time in history, scientists are bringing these fantasies into reality. The free radical theory of aging has provided researchers with a much deeper understanding of the causes of cellular damage and biological aging, as well as how antioxidant nutrients work to prevent or retard this process. As shown in this book, certain drugs and nutrients can produce increases in intelligence, extend life, and slow down the aging process. The dissemination of this information can lead to enormous benefits for all mankind. It is hoped that the research presented in this book will contribute to bringing this important information to the awareness of the general public.

Appendix A
FDA Drug Bulletin: FDA Sanctions "Unapproved" Uses For Drugs

Every month, the U.S. Food and Drug Administration issues an *FDA Drug Bulletin* to provide "information of importance to physicians and other health professionals." These bulletins communicate FDA policy to the medical profession.

The April 1982 issue of the FDA Drug Bulletin included a policy statement of great significance to individuals and health professionals who are interested in intelligence drugs and life extension. The FDA made it clear that *the use of approved drugs for "unapproved" uses is not only legal, but is one of the primary means of therapeutic innovation.*

The FDA encourages physicians to prescribe drugs for unapproved uses in order to provide the best possible health care to the American public. The FDA is to be commended for this enlightened ruling. Physicians who are unaware of this policy decision are often reluctant to write prescriptions for intelligence drugs.

If you would like to reassure your own physician about the legality of prescribing drugs for unapproved uses, just show him or her the FDA policy statement reprinted below:

FDA Drug Bulletin
Policy Statement, April 1982 Issue

"Use of Approved Drugs for Unlabeled Indications"

The appropriateness or the legality of prescribing approved drugs for uses not included in their official labeling is sometimes a cause of concern and confusion among practitioners.

Under the federal Food, Drug, and Cosmetic (FD&C) Act, a drug approved for marketing may be labeled, promoted, and advertised by the manufacturer only for those uses for which the drug's safety and effectiveness have been established and which the FDA has approved. These are commonly referred to as "approved uses." This means that adequate and well-controlled clinical trials have documented these uses, and the results of the trials have been reviewed and approved by the FDA.

The FD&C Act does not, however, limit the manner in which a physician may use an approved drug. Once a product has been approved for marketing, a physician may prescribe it for uses or in treatment regimens or patient populations that are not included in approved labeling. Such "unapproved" uses may be appropriate and rational in certain circumstances, and may, in fact, reflect approaches to drug therapy that have been extensively reported in medical literature.

The term "unapproved uses" is, to some extent, misleading. It includes a variety of situations ranging from unstudied to thoroughly investigated drug uses. Valid new uses for drugs already on the market are often first discovered through serendipitous observations and therapeutic innovations, subsequently confirmed by well-planned and executed clinical investigations. Before such advances can be added to the approved labeling, however, data substantiating the effectiveness of a new use or regimen must be submitted by the manufacturer to the FDA for evaluation. This may take time and, without the initiative of the drug manufacturer whose product is involved, may never occur. For that reason, accepted medical practice often includes drug use that is not reflected in approved drug labeling.

With respect to its role in medical practice, the package insert is informational only. The FDA tries to assure that prescription drug information in the package insert accurately and fully reflects the data on safety and effectiveness on which drug approval is based.

Many physicians are reluctant to prescribe drugs for unapproved uses because they are uncertain of the law regarding this issue. The FDA's ruling suggests that physicians can explore new uses for approved drugs in the course of their practice. This is good news for individuals who want to take advantage of the benefits of intelligence drugs.

Appendix B
Mail Order Medicine

It is a well-known fact that many effective medicines used in many other parts of the world are not available in the United States. Also, new uses for established drugs do not get publicized to doctors or to the general public due to certain FDA policies. Situations like this prevent most Americans from obtaining many substances that could potentially provide great benefit to them. A recent ruling by the FDA has made this problem a little bit easier for people who want to obtain medicines from foreign countries.

The following story was released to and printed in the New York Times on July 25, 1989:

F.D.A. EXPANDS EARLIER STAND BY ALLOWING MAILING OF DRUGS

> When the Food and Drug Administration announced on Saturday that it would allow Americans to import unapproved drugs from abroad in small quantities, it was formalizing its longstanding practice of looking the other way when travelers brought back foreign drugs.
> More significantly, it also stated for the first time that it would permit routine mail shipments of such drugs, making them potentially available to vastly more people than the few who venture abroad in search of treatments.

The following mail order company, Pharmaceuticals International, offers health-oriented pharmaceuticals from around the world. They have a United States mailing address; however, they are located in Mexico and all shipments are sent from Mexico.

Pharmaceuticals International
539 Telegraph Canyon Road
Suite 227
Chula Vista, CA 92010-6492
Telephone: (800) 365-3698

GOT
CATOLOG
5/19/90

Appendix C
Commercial Suppliers

I am frequently asked to recommend sources for the supplements listed in this book. The following companies are not the only sources for these products; however, I have had satisfactory dealings with them and feel comfortable in recommending them. I have no financial connection with any of the following suppliers or any of their products.

> The Life Extension Foundation
> 2835 Hollywood Blvd.
> Hollywood, FL 33020
> Telephone: 1-(800)-841-5433
> In Canada: 1-(800)-826-2114

The Life Extension Foundation carries an extensive line of nutritional supplements as well as life extension products and literature. They also publish an excellent monthly newsletter called *The Life Extension Report*.

> Bronson Pharmaceuticals
> 4526 Rinetti Lane
> La Canada, CA 91011
> Telephone: (818) 790-2646

[handwritten: ✓CATALOG REQUEST 5/10/90 ✓GOT 5/19/90]

This company carries a large selection of nutritional products. Bronson's is an excellent source from which to order bulk quantities of Vitamin C crystals by the pound or kilogram. Mail order only. Write or call for information and order blank mailing envelopes.

Twin Laboratories, Inc.
2120 Smithtown Avenue
Ronkonkoma, NY 11779

TwinLab is one of the largest manufacturers of vitamins and dietary supplements in the United States. Their products are available in many health food stores across the country. They have a product information service and will send out their catalog in response to written requests.

Metagenics, Inc.   *[handwritten: 1 800 638-2848]*
23180 Del Lago
Laguna Hills, CA 92653
Telephone: 1-(800)-692-9400
California: 1-(800)-833-9536

[handwritten: K DISTRIBUTOR ONLY SELLS TO DOCTORS. CALL DIST FF WANT LIST]

Metagenics markets the Mycelized form of Vitamins A and E. They specialize in therapeutic nutritional food supplements and their emphasis is on high-quality formulations, ingredients, vitamins and herbs. All formulas are focused on nutritional support for genetic potential.

Vitamin Research Products
2044-A Old Middlefield Way
Mountain View, CA 94043
Telephone:
In the U.S.A.:   1-(800) 541-1623
In California: 1-(800) 541-8536
In Canada: 1-(800) 225-2896

Vitamin Research offers powdered and crystalline nutritional supplements for manufacturing, processing, or repackaging. Vitamin Research is an inexpensive and reliable source for ordering powdered calcium ascorbate in bulk by the pound or kilogram.

Glossary

Age pigment: a common term used to describe the brown blotchy spots that occur on the skin as a result of aging. Technically these spots are called lipofuscin deposits.

Alpha-tocopherol: the form of vitamin E that has the widest natural distribution in nature and also undergoes the greatest biological activity.

Alzheimer's disease: a form of mental deterioration involving loss of memory and intellectual functions. Other symptoms are apathy, loss of speech, gait disturbances, and disorientation. The disease may take from a few months to four or five years to progress to complete loss of intellectual function.

Antioxidants: a chemical or nutrient that reacts with and neutralizes free radicals. Antioxidants are sometimes called free radical scavengers. Examples of antioxidants are the vitamins A, C, E, some of the B vitamins, beta-carotene, the amino acid cysteine, the trace mineral selenium, the enzyme glutathione peroxidase.

Ascorbic acid: another name for vitamin C.

Ascorbyl Palmitate: a fat-soluble form of vitamin C that exhibits powerful antioxidant properties.

ATP: Adenosine triphosphate. An enzyme found in all cells, but particularly in muscle cells. When this substance is split by enzyme action, energy is produced. The energy of the muscle is stored in this compound.

Auxins: a family of chemicals called plant growth hormones.

Axon: the extension of a nerve cell that conducts impulses away from the cell body.

Beta-carotene: a yellow pigment found in various plant tissues. It is the most biologically active member of the carotene family. Carotenes are the form of vitamin A found in plants and are the precursors of vitamin A in mammals. A liver enzyme splits one molecule of beta-carotene in half, forming two molecules of vitamin A. Beta-carotene is a powerful antioxidant with the special capability of being able to neutralize the singlet oxygen species of free radical.

Bioavailability: the relative amount of a nutrient or drug that is absorbable or available to the body compared to the total amount taken into the body.

Bioflavonoids: a group of compounds that are "cousins" to vitamin C. The main bioflavonoids are hesperidin and rutin. They work synergistically with vitamin C to assist in maintaining a healthy immune system. Classic symptoms of bioflavonoid and vitamin C deficiency are easy bruising and gums that bleed easily when brushing the teeth.

Biological age: the condition or state of health of a person relative to their chronological age.

Bowel tolerance: the amount of vitamin C a person needs to take to saturate their system. At this point water is drawn into the intestines, which softens the consistency of the stools and can cause a diarrhea-like effect.

Calcium ascorbate: the calcium salt of vitamin C. Calcium ascorbate is a less acidic tasting form of vitamin C and it is also a highly absorbable form of calcium.

Carbon monoxide: a gas that has an affinity for the oxygen-carrying site on the hemoglobin molecule that is sixteen times greater than oxygen. Thus, carbon monoxide readily displaces oxygen and can cause hypoxia. Cigarette smoke and automobile exhaust are the two sources of highest exposure to carbon monoxide.

Central nervous system (CNS): that part of the nervous system that contains the brain, spinal cord, and their associated nerves. The CNS includes the parts of the brain governing consciousness and mental activities.

Centrophenoxine: the generic name for the drug Lucidril.

Cerebrovascular insufficiency: a decrease in the amount of blood that reaches the brain due to a narrowing of the blood vessels leading to or in various parts of the brain.

Cerebrospinal fluid: a water/fluid cushion protecting the brain and spinal cord from physical impact.

Cholesterol: a compound produced in the liver and found in high concentrations in animal fats and oils. Cholesterol has many bodily functions. High levels of cholesterol in the blood is statistically related to an increased risk to heart attacks.

Choline: a well-known member of the B vitamin family. One of its main uses is its conversion into the neurotransmitter acetylcholine in the brain (see chapter 7).

Chronological aging: aging measured by the passage of time (minutes, weeks, years, etc.).

Corpus callosum: a bundle of nerve fibers that connects the two hemispheres of the brain.

Cysteine: a sulfur-containing amino acid with antioxidant properties.

D-alpha tocopherol: natural vitamin E.

Deanol: the generic name for DMAE.

DL-alpha tocopherol: synthetic vitamin E, which is less biologically active than natural vitamin E.

Degenerative disease: the gradual deterioration of a biological system resulting from free radical damage.

Dendrites: the fine, tree-like network of extensions that branch out from the body of a nerve cell, and receive impulses and transmit them to the center of the nerve cell.

Diastolic blood pressure: the lower of the two numbers in a blood pressure reading; it is the blood pressure level during the time the heart muscle is relaxed.

Dihydrogenated ergot alkaloids: one of the generic names for the prescription drug Hydergine.

DMAE: the short name for Di-Methyl-Amino-Ethanol. It is a little-known B vitamin that can stimulate the production of acetylcholine. DMAE has also been shown to extend life span in laboratory animals.

DNA: deoxyribonucleic acid, which is the genetic blueprint within the cell of every living organism. Free radical damage to DNA is thought to be directly related to both aging and cancer.

Double-blind: a method of designing a scientific experiment so that neither the experimental subjects nor the investigator knows what treatment, if any, a subject is getting until after the experiment is over. This method of experimental design attempts to eliminate bias from both subjects and investigators.

Engram: the protoplasmic trace of change left by a stimulus in neural tissue.

Enzymes: complex proteins that are capable of inducing chemical changes in other substances without being changed themselves.

Ergoloid mesylates: one of the generic names for the prescription drug Hydergine.

Free radical: a molecule or molecular fragment with a free or unpaired electron. These electrochemically unbalanced structures are very unstable and violently reactive.

Free radical reaction: the self-generating, self-propagating chain reaction of cellular destruction that occurs when a free radical attacks other cells and/or cellular components and goes unchecked. The free radical is trying to gain or capture an extra electron to regain its own electrical stability, but in doing so, it takes electrons away from other molecules, thus creating more free radicals.

Free radical theory of aging: the theory developed by Dr. Denham Harman at the University of Nebraska that postulates that damage by free radicals is the root cause of the damage to biological systems that we know as aging and chronic degenerative disease.

Generic drugs: a drug that is sold under its technical name rather than a single company's brand or trade name. Generic drugs are marketed when the time period on the patent held by the original manufacturer has expired. By law, a generic drug must contain the same ingredients and be at the same strength as the brand name drug for which it is substituted. Generic drugs are usually much less expensive than their brand-name equivalents.

Gerovital: a drug that is widely used throughout Europe in life extension and antiaging therapies. It was developed in Romania by Dr. Ana Aslan.

Glutathione peroxidase: a sulfur-containing enzyme that possesses powerful antioxidant properties. Each molecule of glutathione peroxidase contains four molecules of selenium.

Huntington's disease: a disease of the central nervous system characterized by unusual involuntary movements of the face, arms, and legs and a progressively deteriorating mental state. Onset is usually between thirty and fifty years of age. Treatment with choline and lecithin have occasionally produced partial improvement.

Hydrogenation: a catalyzed chemical reaction whereby hydrogen atoms are forced into the double bond areas of a molecule. This process often changes the geometrical or spatial orientation of the molecule at the double bond site. The hydrogenation process makes fats and oils harmful to the biological systems of animals or humans.

Hypoxia: a condition of partial oxygen deficiency in the blood. During hypoxic conditions, free radical production is greatly increased.

Lecithin: is a compound called phosphatidyl choline. Lecithin is a source of choline that in turn is a precursor for the neurotransmitter acetylcholine in brain chemistry. Lecithin is part of the structural material for every cell in the human body (see Chapter 7).

Lysosomes: subcellular structures that act as the waste disposal units within the cells. Lysosomes contain powerful enzymes to do their digestive waste disposal work. When lysosomal membranes are damaged by free radicals, the lysosomal enzymes leak out and do great harm to the surrounding tissues.

Methionine: a sulfur-containing amino acid with antioxidant properties.

Micelle: a tiny water-soluble cluster of fat manufactured in the small intestine when dietary fat mixes with digestive secretions. The fat-soluble vitamins (A, D, E, and K) and a group of nutrients called the essential fatty acids must be broken down to micelle size before they can be absorbed by the body.

Mitochondria: the "power plants" inside cells where oxygen and nutrients are metabolized to water, carbon dioxide, and energy.

ANTIAGING

Mycelization: a process that reduces nutritional supplements of vitamins A and E down to micelle size. These supplements then require no digestion and have approximately a five times greater rate of absorption than ordinary vitamin A and E supplements.

Nerve: the structure that transmits impulses and stimuli to and from the brain and spinal cord.

Nerve growth factor (NGF): a natural hormone that stimulates the growth of neurites in the brain. There is evidence that Hydergine may also stimulate NGF.

Neuron: a nerve cell, the structural and functional unit of the nervous system.

Neurotransmitter: the chemical messengers that nerve cells use to communicate with each other in the brain.

Nicotine: a poisonous alkaloid found primarily in the leaves of the tobacco plant (and cigarettes). It is one of the most toxic and addictive of all poisons. In the body it causes vasoconstriction that cuts down the amount of blood supply and the amount of oxygen that is able to reach tissues, thus producing hypoxia.

Nootropic: a new class of drugs providing desirable qualities of cerebral stimulation and enhancement without the negative side effects of ordinary psychoactive drugs. The word was coined by Dr. C. Giurgea (Gr.: *noos* = mind; *tropein* = toward).

Oxidation: a type of chemical reaction in which an electron is removed from the compound being oxidized. Removing an electron creates a free radical (a compound lacking an electron or with an unpaired electron). Oxygen is the most common oxidizing compound.

Parkinson's disease: a chronic disease of the central nervous system involving slowly spreading rhythmic tremor, muscular weakness, a peculiar gait, and a mask-like facial expression.

Partially hydrogenated fats: forcing hydrogen to take up some of the double bond sites in unsaturated fats. This gives the fat a longer shelf life commercially, but makes it harmful for animals and humans to eat.

Phosphatidyl choline: a phospholipid (a fat) that the body can use as a precursor to make choline. Phosphatidyl choline is also effective in lowering serum cholesterol.

Piracetam: a drug that exhibits characteristics of enhancing intelligence, memory, and learning as well as slowing down and preventing aspects of brain aging.

Pituitary gland: an endocrine gland located at the base of the brain. It secretes a number of hormones that regulate many bodily processes such as growth, reproduction, and various metabolic activities. It is often called the master gland. Vasopressin is secreted from the pituitary gland.

Placebo: an inactive substance given to satisfy a patient's desire for medicine.

Selenium: an important trace mineral with antioxidant properties. Selenium and antioxidant enzymes containing selenium have shown strong anticancer properties.

Senility: the loss of mental faculties associated with old age.

Singlet oxygen free radical: a single molecule of oxygen that has gained an extra electron. This is a highly reactive state; the singlet oxygen free radical is one of the most destructive free radicals known. Internally, it is a toxic by-product of many metabolic reactions. Smoking is the largest single producer of the singlet oxygen free radical.

Sodium ascorbate: another acid-neutralized (less acidic) form of ascorbic acid.

Stroke: a rupture in a blood vessel in the brain.

Superoxide dismutase (SOD): an antioxidant enzyme containing zinc and copper or manganese. Its main function is to scavenge and neutralize the superoxide free radical.

Synapse: the gap between nerve cells. Chemicals called neurotransmitters are the substances that allow nerves to communicate with each other across the synaptic gaps.

Systolic blood pressure: the higher of the two numbers in a blood pressure reading; it is the force with which blood is pumped when the heart muscle contracts.

Tardive dyskinesia: uncontrollable, slow, rhythmic movements that frequently occur as undesired side effects of therapy with certain psychiatric medications, especially the phenothiazines.

Unsaturated fats: fats that contain double bonds between some of their carbon atoms. These double bond positions are very vulnerable to attack by oxygen and free radicals.

Vasopressin: a brain hormone that is involved with memory, learning, and recall. It also has an antidiuretic effect and is used to elevate blood pressure and retain body fluids in a medical condition called diabetes insipidus (see Chapter 10).

Vitamin A: one of the fat-soluble vitamins and an important antioxidant. Also called retinol, it is the form of vitamin A that is found in animals. It is essential to growth, healthy skin and epithelial tissue, and the prevention of night blindness.

Vitamin C: one of the most important antioxidant nutrients. Also called ascorbic acid, it is essential in building strong, healthy tissue, especially capillary walls.

Vitamin C pump: a biological protective mechanism that steps up the concentration of vitamin C in the spinal fluid ten and in the brain one hundred times greater than the concentration of vitamin C in the circulating blood and body fluids.

Vitamin E: chemically known as d-alpha-tocopherol. Vitamin E is a fat-soluble vitamin and is one of the main antioxidant nutrients. It also promotes fertility and prevents abortion.

Notes

CHAPTER 1: INTRODUCTION

1. Machado, Luis Alberto. *The Right to Be Intelligent*. Elmsford, NY: Pergamon Press, 1980.

CHAPTER 3: MEMORY

1. Kandel, E. R., and H. H. Schwartz. *Principles of Neural Science*. New York: Elsevier-North Holland, 1981.

CHAPTER 4: FREE RADICALS AND ANTIOXIDANTS

1. Harman, Denham. "Free Radical Theory of Aging: Nutritional Implications." *Age*. 1978, Vol. 1, pp. 143–50.
2. Demopoulos, H. B. "The Basis of Free Radical Pathology." *Federation Proceedings*. 1973, Vol. 32, pp. 1859–61.
3. Cranton, E. M., and J. P. Frackelton. "Treatment of Free Radical Pathology in Chronic Degenerative Diseases with EDTA Chelation Therapy." *Journal of Holistic Medicine*. 1984, Vol. 6, No. 1.
4. Demopoulos, H. B., et al. "The Possible role of Free Radical Reactions in Carcinogenesis." *Journal of Environment Pathology and Toxicology*. 1980, Vol. 3, pp. 273–303.
5. Cranton, op. cit.
6. Demopoulos, 1980, op. cit., pp. 273–303.
7. Martin, D. W., et al. *Harper's Review of Biochemistry*. Los Altos, CA: Lange Medical Publications, 1981, p. 129.

CHAPTER 6: INTELLIGENCE, THINKING, AND LEARNING

1. Herrnstein, R. J. *I.Q. in the Meritocracy*. Boston: Little, Brown, 1971, p. 107.
2. Ibid.
3. *Mind Play*, 1987, Vol. 1, No. 1.
4. Diamond, Marian. *Enriching Heredity*. New York: The Free Press, 1988.
5. Ibid.
6. Rosenzveig, Fred. "Can Thinking Be Taught?" *Human Intelligence International Newsletter*. Spring 1987, Vol. 8, No. 1, p. 5.
7. Rico, Gabriel. "Thinking as Patterning." *Human Intelligence International Newsletter*. Winter 1987, Vol. 7, No. 4, p. 4.

8. Brand, Stewart. *The Media Lab*. New York: Viking Penguin, 1987, p. 127.
9. Ibid.
10. Cousins, Norman. "Memories of Bucky." *Saturday Review,* September-October 1983, p. 12.

CHAPTER 7: CHOLINE/LECITHIN

1. Davis, Adelle. *Let's Get Well*. New York: Harcourt Brace Jovanovich, 1965.
2. Gelenberg, Alan, et al. "Lecithin for the Treatment of Tardive Dyskinesia." *Nutrition and the Brain*. 1979, Vol. 5, pp. 285–90.
3. Sitaram, N., and H. Weingartner. "Human Serial Learning: Enhancement with Arecholine and Choline and Impairment with Scopolamine." *Science*. 1978, 201, pp. 275–76.
4. Erasmus, Udo. *Fats and Oils*. Vancouver, Canada: Alive Books, 1986.
5. Werbach, Melvyn. *Nutrition Influences on Illness*. Tarzana, CA: Third Line Press, 1988.
6. Gelenberg, op. cit., pp. 285–90.
7. Pearson, D., and S. Shaw. *Life Extension*. New York: Warner Books, 1982.

CHAPTER 8: DMAE/DEANOL

1. Honegger, Conrad, and Ruth Honegger. "Occurrence and Quantitative Determination of 2-Dimethylaminoethanol in Animal Tissue Extracts." *Nature*. 1959, Vol. 184, pp. 550–52.
2. Pfeiffer, Carl C. "Parasympathetic Neurohumors. Possible Precursors and Effect on Behavior." *International Review of Neurobiology*. 1959, pp. 195–244.
3. Ceder, G., et al. "Effects of 2-Dimethylaminoethanol (Deanol) on the Metabolism of Choline in Plasma." *Journal of Neurochemistry*. 1978, Vol. 30, pp. 1293–96.
4. Pfeiffer, 1959, op. cit., pp. 195–244.
5. Oettinger, Leon. "The Use of Deanol in the Treatment of Disorders of Behavior in Children." *The Journal of Pediatrics*. 1958, Vol. 3, pp. 671–75.
6. Osvaldo Re'. "2-Dimethylaminoethanol (Deanol): A Brief Review of Its Clinical Efficacy and Postulated Mechanism of Action." *Current Therapeutic Research*. 1974, Vol. 16, No. 11, pp. 1238–42.
7. Pfeiffer, Carl C., et al. "Stimulant Effect of 2-Dimethyl-1-aminoethanol: Possible Precursor of Brain Acetylcholine." *Science*. 1957, Vol. 126, pp. 610–11.
8. Pfeiffer, 1959, op. cit., pp. 195–244.
9. Murphree, H. B., et al. "The Stimulant Effect of 2-Diethylaminoethanol (Deanol) in Human Volunteer Subjects." *Clinical Pharmacology and Therapeutics*. 1960, Vol. 1, pp. 303–10.
10. Hochschild, R. "Effect of Dimethylaminoethyl p-Chlorophenoxy-acetate on the Life Span of Male Swiss Webster Albino Mice." *Experimental Gerontology*. 1973, Vol. 8, pp. 177–83.
11. Ibid.

12. Pfeiffer, 1959, op. cit., pp. 195–244.

13. Osvaldo, Re', op. cit., pp. 1238–42.

14. Ibid.

CHAPTER 9: HYDERGINE

1. Exton-Smith, A. N., et al. "Clinical Experience with Ergot Alkaloids." *Aging.* New York: Raven Press, 1983, Vol. 23, p. 323.

2. Hughes, John R., et al. "An Ergot Alkaloid Preparation (Hydergine) in the Treatment of Dementia: A Critical Review of the Clinical Literature." *Journal of the American Geriatrics Society.* 1976, Vol. 24, pp. 490–97.

3. Yoshikawa, Masami, et al. "A Dose-Response Study with Dihydroergotoxine Mesylate in Cerebrovascular Disturbances." *Journal of the American Geriatrics Society.* 1983, Vol. 31, No. 1, pp. 1–7.

4. Rogers, Robert L., et al. "Non-smokers Are Smarter." *Health and Longevity Report.* 1984, Vol. 2, No. 6, p. 8.

5. Emmenegger, H., and W. Meier-Ruge. "The Actions of Hydergine on the Brain." *Pharmacology.* 1968, Vol. 1, pp. 65–78.

6. Copeland, R. L., Jr., et al. "Behavioral and Neurochemical Effects of Hydergine in Rats." *Archives of International Pharmacodynamics.* 1981, Vol. 252, pp. 113–23.

7. Rao, Dodda B., and John R. Norris. "A Double-Blind Investigation of Hydergine in the Treatment of Cerebrovascular Insufficiency in the Elderly." *Johns Hopkins Medical Journal.* 1971, Vol. 130, pp. 317–23.

8. Weil, C., ed. "Pharmacology and Clinical Pharmacology of Hydergine." *Handbook of Experimental Pharmacology.* New York: Springer-Verlag, 1978.

9. Nandy, K., and F. H. Schneider. "Effects of Dihydroergotoxine Mesylate on Aging Neurons in vitro." *Gerontology.* 1978, Vol. 24, pp. 66–70.

10. Ibid.

11. Yesavage, Jerome A., et al. "Dihydroergotoxine: 6-Mg versus 3-Mg Dosage in the Treatment of Senile Dementia. Preliminary Report." *Journal of the American Geriatrics Society.* 1979, Vol. 27, No. 2, pp. 80–82.

12. Fanchamps, Albert. "Dihydroergotoxine in Senile Cerebral Insufficiency." *Aging.* New York: Raven Press, 1983, Vol. 23, pp. 311–22.

13. Hindmarch, I., et al. "The Effects of an Ergot Alkaloid Derivative (Hydergine) on Aspects of Psychomotor Performance, Arousal, and Cognitive Processing Ability." *The Journal of Clinical Pharmacology.* November-December 1979, pp. 726–31.

14. Spiegel, Rene, et al. "A Controlled Long-Term Study with Ergoloid Mesylates (Hydergine) in Healthy, Elderly Volunteers: Results After Three Years." *Journal of the Geriatrics Society.* 1983, Vol. 31, No. 9, pp. 549–55.

15. Kleimola, Terttu. "Generic Bioavailability Test." Turku, Finland: Leiras Pharmaceuticals, 1982.

CHAPTER 10: VASOPRESSIN/DIAPID

1. Gold, Philip W., et al. "Effects of 1-Desamo-8-Arginine Vasopressin on Behavior and Cognition in Primary Affective Disorders." *The Lancet.* November 10, 1979, pp. 992–94.

2. De Wied, D., et al. "Vasopressin and Memory Consolidation." *Perspectives in Brain Research*. New York: Elsevier Scientific Publishing, 1975.

3. Oliveros, J. C., et al. "Vasopressin in Amnesia." *The Lancet*. January 7, 1978, p. 42.

4. Legros, J. J., et al. "Influence of Vasopressin on Learning and Memory." *The Lancet*. January 7, 1978, pp. 41–42.

5. Gold, op. cit., pp. 992–94.

6. Oliveros, op. cit., p. 42.

7. Legros, op. cit., pp. 41–42.

8. Laczi, F., et al. "Effects of Lysine-Vasopressin and 1-Deamino-8-D-Arginine-Vasopressin on Memory in Healthy Individuals and Diabetes Insipidus Patients." *Psychoneuroendocrinology*. 1982, Vol. 7, No. 2, pp. 185–92.

9. Legros, op. cit., pp. 41–42.

10. Pearson, D., and S. Shaw. *Life Extension*. New York: Warner Books, 1982.

Chapter 11: Lucidril

1. Mann, D. M. "A and E." *Science*. 1981, Vol. 214, pp. 640–41.

2. Jarvik, L. F. "The Aging Nervous System: Clinical Aspects." *Aging*. New York: Raven Press, 1975, Vol. 1, pp. 1–9.

3. Nandy, K. "Aging Neurons and Pharmacological Agents." *Aging*. New York: Raven Press, 1983, Vol. 21, pp. 401–15.

4. Demopoulos, H. B., et al. "Molecular Pathology of Lipids in CNS Membranes." *Oxygen & Physiological Function*. 1977, pp. 491–508.

5. Nandy, K., and G. H. Bourne. "Effect of Centrophenoxine on the Lipofuscin Pigments of the Neurones of Senile Guinea Pigs." *Nature*. 1966, Vol. 210, pp. 313–14.

6. Riga, S., and D. Riga. "Effects of Centrophenoxine on the Lipofuscin Pigments of the Nervous System of Old Rats." *Brain Research*. 1974, Vol. 72, pp. 265–75.

7. Nandy, K. "Lipofuscinogenesis in Mice Early Treated with Centrophenoxine." *Mechanisms of Aging and Development*. 1978, Vol. 8, pp. 131–38.

8. Giuli, D., et al. "Morphometric Studies on Synapses of the Cerebellar Glomerulus: The Effect of Centrophenoxine Treatment in Old Rats." *Mechanisms of Aging and Development*. 1980, Vol. 14, pp. 265–71.

9. Marcer, D., and S. M. Hopkins. "The Differential Effects of Meclofenoxate on Memory Loss in the Elderly." *Age and Aging*. 1977, Vol. 6, pp. 123–31.

10. Hochschild, R. "Effect of Dimethylaminoethyl p-Chlorophenoxy-acetate on the Life Span of Male Swiss Webster Albino Mice." *Experimental Gerontology*. 1973, Vol. 8, pp. 177–83.

11. Giuli, op. cit., pp. 265–71.

Chapter 12: Dilantin/DPH

1. Reznick, O. "The Psychoactive Properties of Diphenylhydantoin: Experiences with Prisoners and Juvenile Delinquents." *International Journal of Neuropsychiatry*. 1967, Vol. 3, pp. 30–48.

2. Ibid., pp. 30–48.

3. Dreyfus, J. J., Jr. "The Beneficial Effects of Diphenylhydantoin on the Nervous System of Nonepileptics—As Experienced and Observed in Others by a Layman." Presented at the American College of Neuropsychopharmacology, December 7, 1966. *Dreyfus Medical Foundation*. 1966.

4. Smith, W. L., and J. B. Lowrey. "Effects of Diphenylhydantoin on Mental Abilities in the Elderly." *Journal of the American Geriatrics Society*. 1975, Vol. 23, No. 5, pp. 207–11.

5. Haward, L. R. C. "Effects of Sodium Diphenylhydanoinate and Pemoline Upon Concentration: A Comparative Study." *Drugs and Cerebral Function*. 1970, pp. 103–20.

6. Smith, W. L., and J. B. Lowrey. "The Effects of Diphenylhydantoin on Cognitive Functions in Man." *Drugs, Development, and Cerebral Function*. 1972, pp. 344–51.

7. Smith, W. L., and J. B. Lowrey. "Effects of Diphenylhydantoin on Mental Abilities in the Elderly." *Journal of the American Geriatrics Society*. 1975, Vol. 23, No. 5, pp. 207–11.

8. Gordon, P. "Diphenylhydantoin and Procainamide Normalization of Suboptimal Learning Behavior." *Recent Advances in Biological Psychiatry*. 1968, Vol. 10, pp. 121–33.

9. Doty, B., and R. Dalman. "Diphenylhydantoin Effects of Avoidance Condition As a Function of Age and Problem Difficulty." *Psychosocial Science*, 1969, Vol. 14, pp. 109–11.

CHAPTER 13: COGNITIVE ENHANCERS

1. Poschel, B. P. H. "New Pharmacologic Perspectives on Nootropic Drugs." *Handbook of Psychopharmacology*. 1988, pp. 11–18.

2. Bylinsky, Gene. "Medicine's Next Marvel: The Memory Pill." *Fortune*. January 20, 1986, pp. 68–72.

3. DeNoble, Victor, et al. "Vinpocetine: Nootropic Effects on Scopolamine-Induced and Hypoxia-Induced Retrieval Deficits of a Step-Through Passive Avoidance Response in Rats." *Pharmacology Biochemistry & Behavior*. 1986, Vol. 24, pp. 1123–28.

4. Otomo, E., et al. "Comparison of Vinpocetine with Ifenprodil Tartrate and Dihydroergotoxine Mesylate Treatment and Results of Long-Term Treatment with Vinpocetine." *Current Therapeutic Research*. 1985, Vol. 37, No. 5, pp. 811–21.

5. Hadjiev, D. and S. Yancheva. "Rheoencephalographic and Psychologic Studies with Ethyl Apovincaminate in Cerebral Vascular Insufficiency." *Arzneimittelforschung*. 1976, Vol. 26, pp. 1947–50.

6. Subhan, Z., and I. Hindmarch. "Psychopharmacological Effects of Vinpocetine in Normal Healthy Volunteers." *European Journal of Clinical Pharmacology*. 1985, Vol. 28, pp. 567–71.

7. DeNoble, op. cit., pp. 1123–28.

8. Cumin, R., et al. "Effects of the Novel Compound Aniracetam (Ro

13-5057) Upon Impaired Learning and Memory in Rodents." *Psychopharmacology*. 1982, Vol. 78, pp. 104–11.

9. Vincent, George, et al. "The Effects of Aniracetam (Ro-13-5057) on the Enhancement and Protection of Memory." *Annals of the New York Academy of Sciences*. 1985, Vol. 244, pp. 489–91.

10. Cumin, op. cit., pp. 104–11.

11. Murry, C. L., and H. C. Fibiger. "The Effect of Pramiracetam (CI-879) on the Acquisition of a Radial Arm Maze Task." *Psychopharmacology*. 1986, Vol. 89, pp. 378–81.

12. Poschel, op. cit., pp. 11–18.

13. Dejong, Richard. "Safety of Pramiracetam." *Current Therapeutic Research*. February 1987, Vol. 41, No. 2, pp. 254–57.

14. Wilsher, Colin R. "Piracetam and Dyslexia: Effects on Reading Tests." *Journal of Clinical Psychopharmacology*. 1987, Vol. 7, No. 4, pp. 230–37.

15. Itil, R. M., et al. "CNS Pharmacology and Clinical Therapeutic Effects of Oxiracetam." *Clinical Neuropharmacology*. 1986, Vol. 9, Supp. 3. New York: Raven Press, pp. S70–S78.

16. Pellegata, R., et al. "Cyclic Gaba-Gabob Analogues." Presented at *VI International Meeting of the International Society For Neurochemistry*, Copenhagen, August 21–26, 1977.

17. Mondadori, C., et al. "Effects of Oxiracetam on Learning and Memory in Animals: Comparison with Piracetam." *Clinical Neuropharmacology*. 1986, Vol. 9, Supp. 13. New York: Raven Press, pp. S27–S37.

18. Ferrero, Enrico. "Controlled Clinical Trial of Oxiracetam in the Treatment of Chronic Cerebrovascular Insufficiency in the Elderly. *Current Therapeutic Research*. August 1984, Vol. 36, No. 2, pp. 298–308.

19. Ammassari-Teule, M., et al. "Avoidance Facilitation in Adult Mice by Prenatal Administration of the Nootropic Drug Oxiracetam." *Pharmacological Research Communications*. 1986, Vol. 18, No. 12, pp. 1169–78.

20. Poschel, op. cit., pp. 11-18.

CHAPTER 14: PIRACETAM

1. Giurgea, C. E. "The 'Nootropic' Approach to the Pharmacology of the Integrative Activity of the Brain." *Conditional Reflex*. 1973, Vol. 8, No. 2, pp. 108–15.

2. Dimond, S. J., and E. Y. M. Browers. "Increase in the Power of Human Memory in Normal Man Through the Use of Drugs." *Psychopharmacology*. 1976, Vol. 49, pp. 307–9.

3. Giurgea, C. E., and M. Salama. "Nootropic Drugs." *Progress in Neuropsychopharmacology*. 1977, Vol. 1, pp. 235–47.

4. Mindus, P., et al. "Piracetam-Induced Improvement of Mental Performance: A Controlled Study on Normally Aging Individuals."*ACTA Psychiatrica Scandinavia*. 1976, Vol. 54, pp. 150–60.

5. Buresova, O., and J. Bures. "Piracetam-Induced Facilitation of Interhemispheric Transfer of Visual Information in Rats." *Psychopharmacologia* (Berlin). 1976, Vol. 46, pp. 93–102.

6. Giurgea, C. E. "A Drug for the Mind." *Chemtech*. June 1980, pp. 360–65.

7. Dimond, op. cit., pp. 307–9.

8. Nickerson, V. J., and O. L. Wolthuis. "Effect of the Acquisition-Enhancing Drug Piracetam on Rat Cerebral Energy Metabolism Comparison with Naftidrofuryl and Methamphetamine." *Biochemical Pharmacology*. 1976, Vol. 25, pp. 2241–44.

9. Ibid.

10. Bartus, Raymond T., et al. "Profound Effects of Combining Choline and Piracetam on Memory Enhancement and Cholinergic Function in Aged Rats." *Neurobiology of Aging*. 1981, Vol. 2, pp. 105–11.

11. U.B.C. Laboratories, Pharmaceutical Division. "Basic Scientific and Clinical Data of Nootropil." Brussels, Belgium: U.B.C. Laboratories, 1977.

12. Wilsher, Colin R., et al. "Piracetam and Dyslexia: Effects on Reading Tests." *Journal of Clinical Psychopharmacology*. 1987, Vol. 7, No. 4, pp. 230–37.

13. Dilanni, M., et al. "The Effects of Piracetam in Children with Dyslexia." *Journal of Clinical Psychopharmacology*. 1985, Vol. 5, pp. 272–78.

14. Chase, C. H. et al. "A New Chemotherapeutic Investigation: Piracetam Effects on Dyslexia." *Annals of Dyslexia*. 1984, Vol. 34, pp. 29–48.

15. Conners, et al. "Piracetam and Event-Related Potentials in Dyslexic Children." *Psychopharmacology Bulletin*. 1984, Vol. 20, pp. 667–73.

16. Giurgea, 1973, op. cit., pp. 108–15.

17. Giurgea, 1973, op. cit., pp. 108–15.

18. Steglink, A. J. "The Clinical Use of Piracetam, a New Nootropic Drug." *Arzneimittelforschung*. 1972, Vol. 22, No. 6, pp. 975–77.

19. Donaldson, Thomas. "Therapies to Improve Memory." *Anti-Aging News*. 1984, No. 4, pp. 13-21.

CHAPTER 15: PIRACETAM + CHOLINE

1. Bartus, Raymond T., et al. "Profound Effects of Combining Choline and Piracetam on Memory Enhancement and Cholinergic Function in Aged Rats." *Neurobiology of Aging*. March 1981, pp. 105–11.

2. Friedman, E., et al. "Clinical Response to Choline Plus Piracetam in Senile Dementia: Relation to Red-Cell Choline Levels." *The New England Journal of Medicine*. 1981, 304, No. 24, pp. 1490–91.

3. Kent, Saul. "Piracetam Increases Brain Energy." *Anti-Aging News*. 1981, Vol. 2, No. 10, pp. 65–69.

4. Bartus, op. cit.

5. Ibid.

6. Ferris, S. H., et al. "Combination of Choline/Piracetam in the Treatment of Senile Dementia." *Psychopharmacology Bulletin*. 1982, Vol. 18, pp. 94–98.

7. Poschel, B. P. H. "New Pharmacologic Perspectives on Nootropic Drugs." *Handbook of Psychopharmacology*, 1988, pp. 24–25.

8. Parducz, A. "Depletion of Synaptic Vesicle Lipids in Stimulated Cholinergic Nerve Terminals." *Alzheimer's Disease: Advances in Basic Research and Therapies*. Proceedings of the Third Meeting of the International Study Group of

the Treatment of Memory Disorders Associated with Aging, Zürich, Switzerland, 1984, pp. 217–26.

9. Wurtman, R. J., et al. "Piracetam Diminishes Hippocampal Acetylcholine Levels in Rats." *Life Science*. 1981, Vol. 28, pp. 1091–93.

CHAPTER 16: THE HERBAL WAY

1. Lust, John. *The Herb Book*. New York: Bantam Books, 1974, p. 4.

2. Mowrey, Daniel B. *The Scientific Validation of Herbal Medicine*. Lehi, Utah: Cormorant Books, 1986.

3. Ibid., pp. 191–94.

CHAPTER 17: GINKGO BILOBA

1. Auguet, M., et al. "Bases Pharmacologiques de l'Impact Vasculaire de l'Extrait de *Ginkgo Biloba*," *La Presse Medicale*. 1986, Vol. 15, No. 31, p. 1524.

2. Taillandier, J., et al. "Traitement des Troubles vu Viellissement Cerebral par l'Extrait de *Ginkgo Biloba*." *La Presse Medicale*. 1986, Vol. 15, No. 31. p. 1583.

3. *La Presse Medicale*. 1986, Vol. 15, No. 31, p. 1562.

4. "Anti-radical Properties of *Ginkgo Biloba* Extract." *La Presse Medicale*. 1986, Vol. 15, No. 31, p. 1475.

5. Schaffler, K., and P. Reeh, "Long-term Drug Administration Effects of *Ginkgo Biloba* on the Performance of Healthy Subjects Exposed to Hypoxia." From Agnoli, J., *Effects of Ginkgo Biloba Extracts on Organic Cerebral Impairment*. Eurotext Ltd., 1985, pp. 77–84.

6. Hindmarch, I. "Activity of *Ginkgo Biloba* Extract on Short-term Memory." *La Presse Medicale*. 1986, Vol. 15, No. 31, p. 1592.

7. Gebner, A., et al. "Study of the Long-term Action of a *Ginkgo Biloba* Extract on Vigilance and Mental Performance as Determined by Means of Quantitative Pharmaco-EEG and Psychometric Measurements." *Arzneimittelforschung*. Vol. 35, No. 9, p. 1459.

8. Warburton, D. M. "Clinical Psychopharmacology of *Ginkgo Biloba* Extract." *La Presse Medicale*. 1986, Vol. 15, No. 31, p. 1595.

9. Allard, M. "Treatment of Old Age Disorders with *Ginkgo Biloba* Extract." *La Presse Medicale*. 1986, Vol. 15, No. 31, p. 1540.

CHAPTER 18: GINSENG

1. "Ginseng: The Anti-Stress Therapy." *Anti-Aging News*. October 1983, p. 111.

2. Donsbach, Kurt, and Walter Ziglar. *Ginseng*. Huntington Beach, CA: The International Institute of Natural Health Sciences, 1981, p. 10.

3. Petkov, V. "Effects of Standardized Ginseng Extract on Learning, Memory, and Physical Capabilities." *American Journal of Chinese Medicine*. 1987, Vol. 15, No. 1, pp. 19–29.

4. Baburin, E. F. "On the Effect of *Eleutherococcos senticosus* on the Results of Work and Hearing Acuity of Radio-Telegraphers." In I. I. Brekhman, ed., *Eleutherococcus and Other Adaptogens Among the Far Eastern Plants*. Vladivostok, U.S.S.R.: Far Eastern Publishing House. 1966, pp. 179–84.

5. Donsbach, op. cit., p. 10.

6. Quiroga, H. A., and A. E. Imbriano. "The Effect of Panax Ginseng Extract on Cerebrovascular Deficits." *Orientacion Medica*. 1979, Vol. 28: 1208, pp. 86–87.

7. Petkov, V. *Pharmazeutische Zeitung*. 1968, Vol. 31.

8. *Anti-Aging News*, op. cit., p. 117.

9. Iljutjecok, R. Ju., and S. R. Tjaplygina. "The Effect of a Preparation of *Eleutherococcus Senticosus* on Memory in Mice." The Department of Physiology, Academy of Sciences of the Soviet Union, Novosibirsk, 1978.

10. Simon, Walther C. M. "Efficiency Control of a Gero-Therapeutic Containing Ginseng by Means of Kraepelin's Working Test." *Proceedings of the International Gerontological Symposium Singapore*. February 1977, pp. 199–206.

11. *Anti-Aging News*, op. cit., p. 112.

12. Donsbach, 1981, op. cit., pp. 17–18.

13. Brekham, I. I. *Eleutherococcus*. Leningrad: Nauka Publishing House, 1968.

14. Kamen, Betty. *Siberian Ginseng*. New Canaan, CT: Keats Publishing. 1988, p. 2.

15. Voskersarsky, T. A. Devytkine, et al. "Effect of Eleutherococcus and Ginseng of the Development of Free-Radical Pathology." *Proceeding of the Second International Symposium of Eleutherococcus*. Moscow, 1985, pp. 141–45.

16. Petkov, V., and S. Staneua. "The Effect of an Extract of Ginseng on the Adrenal Cortex." *Proceedings of the 2nd International Pharmacology Meeting*. Prague, 1963. New York: Pergamon Press. Vol. 7, pp. 39–45.

17. Wang, et al. *Advances in Chinese Medical Materials*. 1985, pp. 519–27.

18. Fulder, S. "The Drug That Builds Russians." *New Scientist*, 1980.

19. Kamen, op. cit., p. 12.

20. *Ginseng, Ten of the Most Commonly Asked Questions About the Root of Life*. International Health Publications, 1977 (pamphlet).

21. Seigel, R. D. "Ginseng Abuse Syndrome." *Journal of the American Medical Association*. 1979.

CHAPTER 19: INTRODUCTION TO ANTIAGING

1. Dean, Ward. *Biological Aging Measurement, Clinical Applications*. Los Angeles: The Center for Bio-Gerontology, October 1988.

2. Bland, Jeffrey. *Metabolic Update*. Gig Harbor, WA: HealthComm, 1988.

CHAPTER 20: OPTIMAL NUTRITION AND INTELLIGENCE

1. Benton, David, and Gwilym Roberts. "Effect of Vitamin and Mineral Supplementation on Intelligence of a Sample of School Children. *The Lancet*, January 23, 1988, pp. 140–43.

2. Schoenthaler, Stephen J., et al. "The Impact of a Low Food Additive and Sucrose Diet on Academic Performance in 803 New York City Public Schools." *International Journal of Biosocial Research*, 1986, Vol. 8, No. 2, pp. 185–95.

3. Williams, R. *Nutrition Against Disease*. New York: Bantam Books, 1971.

4. Eaton, Boyd S., and Melvin Konner. "Paleolithic Nutrition." *The New England Journal of Medicine*. 1985, Vol. 312, No. 5, pp. 283–89.

CHAPTER 21: VITAMIN C/ASCORBIC ACID

1. Cranton, E. M., and J. P. Frackelton. "Treatment of Free Radical Pathology in Chronic Degenerative Diseases with EDTA Chelation Therapy." *Journal of Holistic Medicine*. 1984, Vol. 6, No. 1.

2. Ibid.

3. Lesser, Michael. *Nutrition and Vitamin Therapy*. New York: Bantam Books, 1980, pp. 75–76.

4. Cathcart, Robert. "Vitamin C, Titrating to Bowel Tolerance, Anascorbemia and Acute Induced Scurvy." *Medical Hypothesis*. 1981, Vol. 7, p. 1361.

5. Pauling, Linus. *Vitamin C, The Common Cold & The Flu*. San Francisco: W. H. Freeman, 1970.

CHAPTER 22: SELENIUM

1. Bland, Jeffrey. *Diagnostic Usefulness of Trace Elements in Human Hair*. Bellevue, WA: Northwest Diagnostic Services, 1981. p. 22.

2. Lesser, Michael. *Nutrition and Vitamin Therapy*. New York: Bantam Books, 1980, p. 149.

3. Levine, Stephen A. *Antioxidant Biochemical Adaptation*. San Francisco: Biocurrent Research Corporation, 1984.

4. Jackson, M. L. "Selenium: Geochemical Distribution and Associations with Human Heart and Cancer Death Rates and Longevity in China and the United States." *Selenium, Present Status and Perspectives in Biology and Medicine*. NJ: Humana Press, 1987.

5. Passwater, Richard. *Selenium as Food and Medicine*. New Canaan, CT: Keats Publishing, 1980.

6. Chen, L. H. "Effect of Vitamin E and Selenium on Tissue Antioxidant Status of Rats." *Journal of Nutrition*. 1987, Vol. 103, pp. 503–8.

7. McConnell, K. P., and G. J. Cho. "Active Transport of Selenmethionine in the Intestine." *American Journal of Physiology*. 1967, Vol. 45.

8. Wolfram, S., et al. "In Vivo Intestinal Absorption of Selenate and Selenite by Rats." *Journal of Nutrition*. 1985, Vol. 45.

9. Schrauzer, G. N., and D. A. White. "Selenium in Human Nutrition: Dietary Intakes and Effects of Supplementation." *Bioinorganic Chemistry*, 1978, Vol. 8, pp. 303–18.

10. Passwater, op. cit., p. 134.

11. Schrauzer, G. N. "Effects of Temporary Selenium Supplementation on the Genesis of Spontaneous Mammary Tumors in Inbred Female C3H/St Mice." *Carcinogensis*. 1980, Vol. 1, pp. 199–201.

Chapter 23: Vitamin E

1. Harman, D. *Journal of Gerontology*. Vol. 12, pp. 257–63.
2. Martin, D., et al. *Harper's Review of Biochemistry*. 18th ed. Los Altos, CA: Lange Medical Publications, 1981.
3. Scott, Milton L. "Advances on Our Understanding of Vitamin E." *Federation Proceedings 39*, No. 10. 1980, pp. 2736–39.
4. Lesser, Michael. *Nutrition and Vitamin Therapy*. New York: Bantam Books, 1980, p. 100.
5. Bland, Jeffrey. *Metabolic Update*. Metabolic Update tape series. February 1982, Bellevue, WA.
6. Passwater, Richard. *Super-Nutrition*. New York: Simon and Schuster, 1975.
7. Gerras, C., ed. *The Complete Book of Vitamins*. Emmaus, PA: Rodale Press, 1977.
8. Bland, Jeffrey. "New Nutrient Delivery Systems Part 3." *Anabolism*. 1983, Vol. 2, No. 8, pp. 5–6.
9. Briggs, Michael, and Maxine Briggs. "Vitamin E and Oral Contraceptives." *American Journal of Clinical Nutrition*. May 1975.
10. Werbach, Melvyn R. *Nutritional Influence on Illness*. CA: Third Line Press, 1988, p. 464.
11. Passwater, op. cit.
12. Bland, Jeffrey. *Review of Molecular Medicine Vol 1*. Gig Harbor, WA: JSB and Associates, 1985, p. 215.

Chapter 24: Vitamin A/Beta-Carotene

1. Petro, R., et al. "Can Dietary Beta-carotene Materially Reduce Human Cancer Rates?" *Nature*. 1981, Vol. 290, p. 201–7.
2. Levin, Stephen A., and Jeffrey H. Reinhardt, "Biochemical-Pathology Initiated by Free Radicals, Oxidant Chemicals, and Therapeutic Drugs in the Etiology of Chemical Hypersensitivity Disease." *The Journal of Orthomolecular Psychiatry*. 1983, Vol. 12, No. 3, pp. 166–83.
3. Davis, Adelle. *Let's Get Well*. New York: Harcourt Brace Jovanovich. 1965, pp. 313.

Chapter 25: Gerovital/GH-3

1. Bailey, Herbert. *GH-3*. New York: Bantam Books. 1977, pp. 284–85.
2. Advertising Flyer. Dr. Charles Atkins, Ontario, Canada.
3. Aslan, Anna, et al. "Long-term Treatment with Procaine (Gerovital-H3) in Albino Rats." *Journal of Gerontology*. 1965, Vol. 20, p. 1.
4. Verzar, Frederick. "Note on the Influence of Procaine, PABA, and DEAE on the Aging of Rats." *Gerontologia*. 1959, Vol. 3, p. 351.
5. Samorajski, T., and C. Rolstein. "Effects of Chronic Dosage with Chlorpromazine and Gerovital-H3 in the Aging Brain." *Aging Brain & Senile Dementia*. New York: Plenum Press, 1976.

6. Aslan, Anna. "The Therapeutics of Old Age—the Action of Procaine." Blumenthal, H. T., ed., *Medical and Clinical Aspects of Aging*. New York: Columbia University Press, 1962.

7. Smigel, J. O., et al. "H3 (Procaine Hydrochloride) Therapy in Aging Institutionalized Patients: An Interim Report." *Journal of American Gerontological Society*. 1960, Vol. 8, p. 785.

8. Bailey, op. cit., p. 37.

9. "Gerovital-H3: The Youth Drug." *Anti-Aging News*. January 1981, p. 2.

10. Ibid.

11. Zwerling, I. "Effects of a Procaine Preparation (Gerovital-H3) in Hospitalized Geriatric Patients—a Double Blind Study." *Journal of American Gerontological Society*. Vol. 23, p. 8.

12. *Anti-Aging News*, op. cit., p. 2.

13. Ibid.

14. Walford, Roy L. *Maximum Life Span*. New York: W. W. Norton, 1983.

15. Bai, F., R. Michel, and P. Rossignol. *Mech Ageing Development*. 1984, Vol. 26, pp. 277–82.

16. Ostfeld, Adrian, et al. "The Systemic Use of Procaine in the Treatment of the Elderly: A Review." *Journal of the American Geriatrics Society*. January 1977, Vol. 25, pp. 1–19.

17. Thomas, Richard. "Procaine. Will It Keep You Younger Longer?" *The Medical Journal of Australia*. June 11, 1983, pp. 543–45.

18. Bailey, op. cit., p. 168.

19. Product insert. Intreprinderea de Medicamente Bucuresti.

CHAPTER 26: EXERCISE AND THE MIND

1. Bortz, Walter M. "Disuse and Aging." *JAMA*. 1982, Vol. 248, No. 10, pp. 1203–7.

2. De Coverly Veale, D. M. W. "Exercise and Mental Health." *Acta Psychiatry Scandinavia*. 1987, Vol. 76, pp. 113–20.

3. Fellman, Bruce. "Exercise Your Way to Happiness." *Prevention*. May 1981, pp. 68–73.

4. Dustman, Robert E. "Aerobic Exercise Training and Improved Neuropsychological Function of Older Individuals." *Neurobiology of Aging*. 1984, Vol. 5, pp. 35–42.

5. Harris, Gardiner. "The Benefits and Risks of Exercise." *Complementary Medicine*. 1988, pp. 6–11.

6. Samorajski, Thaddeus. "International Congress of Biomedical Gerontology Conference Report." Fahy, Gregory. *Anti-Aging News*. 1985, p. 135.

7. Bortz, op. cit., pp. 1203–7.

CHAPTER 27: FATS AND OILS AND THE BRAIN

1. Erasmus, Udo. *Fats and Oils*. Vancouver, Canada: Alive Books. 1986, p. 42.

2. Rudin, Donald, and Clara Felix, et al. *The Omega-3 Phenomenon*. New York: Rawson Associates. 1987, p. 20.

3. Erasmus, Udo. *Fats That Heal, Fats That Kill*. Vancouver, Canada: Designing Health. 1988, pp. 12–14.

4. Fusco, Carmen L. "Ask Anti-Aging News." *Anti-Aging News*. June 1983, p. 72.

5. Erasmus, *Fats That Heal, Fats That Kill*, pp. 3–4.

6. Rudin, op. cit., p. 19.

7. Erasmus, *Fats and Oils*, pp. 42–43.

8. Erasmus, *Fats That Heal, Fats That Kill*, p. 15.

9. Passwater, Richard. *EPA-Marine Lipids*. New Canaan, CT: Keats Publishing, 1982.

10. Erasmus, *Fats That Heal, Fats That Kill*, pp. 11–12.

11. Passwater, Richard. *Evening Primrose Oil*. New Canaan, CT: Keats Publishing, 1981.

Chapter 29: The Aging Brain

1. Henig, Robin Marantz. *The Myth of Senility*. Washington, DC: AARP, p. 60.

2. Birren, James E., et al. *Human Aging I: A Biological and Behavioral Study*. Washington, DC: U.S. Government Printing Office, 1974.

3. Henig, op. cit., pp. 46–47.

4. American Psychiatric Association Task Force on Nomenclature and Statistics (1952). *Diagnostic and Statistical Manual of Mental Disorders* (DSM-III) 3rd ed., Washington, DC: American Psychiatric Association, pp. 124–26.

5. Kahn, Robert. "Memory Complaint and Impairment in the Aged: The Effect of Depression and Altered Brain Function." *Archives of General Psychiatry*, December 1975, Vol. 32, pp. 1,569–73.

6. Katzman, Robert, et al. "Advances in the Diagnosis of Dementia: Accuracy of Diagnosis and Consequences of Misdiagnosis of Disorders Causing Dementia." *Aging and the Brain*, ed. by R. D. Terry. New York: Raven Press, 1988.

7. Ibid.

8. Watkin, Donald M. "Certain Aspects of the Effect of Age on the Acquisition of Nutrients." *Nutrition in Gerontology*, ed. by J. M. Ordy. New York: Raven Press, 1984.

9. Katzman, op. cit.

10. Morgan, L. G., and Roberta Morgan. *Brainfood: Nutrition and Your Brain*. Tucson, AZ: The Body Press, 1987, pp. 285–95.

11. Stone, Irwin. "Ascorbic Acid Therapy for Aging & Alzheimer's Disease." *Anti-Aging News*. May 1983, p. 51

12. Reisberg, Barry. "An Overview of Current Concepts of Alzheimer's Disease, Senile Dementia, and Age-Associated Cognitive Decline." *Alzheimer's Disease*. New York: Free Press, 1983.

13. Tennant, Forest S., Jr. "Preliminary Observations on Naltrexone for Treatment of Alzheimer's Type Dementia." *Journal of the American Geriatrics Society*, April 1987, Vol. 35, No. 4, pp. 369–70.

14. Tennant, Forest S., Jr. *Preventive Medicine Update*. Gig Harbor, WA: HealthComm, Inc., January 1989.

15. Bland, Jeffrey S. *Review of Molecular Medicine*. Gig Harbor, WA: J.S.B. & Associates, Inc., 1985, Vol. I, p. 86.

16. Ibid., p. 85.

17. Stone, Irwin. "The Most Misunderstood Epidemic Disease in 20th Century Medicine." Talk presented at the National Health Federation, June 26, 1982, San Jose, CA. Reprint No. 120-T from the IS-FACT Foundation.

18. Stone, Irwin. "Ascorbic Acid Therapy for Aging & Alzheimer's Disease." *Anti-Aging News*. May 1983, p. 51

19. Hutton, J. Thomas. "Alzheimer's Disease: Evolving Clinical Concepts and Management Strategies." *Comprehensive Therapy*. 1987, Vol. 13 (9), pp. 55–64.

20. Thomas, L. "On the Problem of Dementia." *Discover*. 1981, Vol. 2, No. 34.

Acknowledgments

This has been an exciting project and we would like to extend special thanks to several people who have given of their time, energy, and friendship to help bring this book to completion. We gratefully acknowledge:

Dr. Ward Dean, for his professional contributions, personal interest, and support. His knowledge and leadership in the fields of life extension and biogerontology have been a source of inspiration and guidance.

Lee Overholser, for his organizational and editing skills, for his generous commitment and great brain, and for being the coach and backbone of this book.

Janie Wilkinson, for tireless proofreading, editing, friendship, and undying support.

Our great friends Mimmie Lewis and Sam Holt, for hours of editing, great suggestions, and sharing the excitement of this project.

Loren Israelsen, Dr. Dan Mowrey, Dr. Gerhard Schrauzer, Dr. Udo Erasmus, Peter Finkle, and Paul Sitt for lending their generous professional expertise, reviewing chapters, and providing research.

To our parents, Ginny and Monte Pelton and Joanne and Oscar Clarke, for planting the seeds of curiosity and the desire to maximize our potential.

Ross Pelton graduated from the University of Wisconsin with a degree in Pharmacy. He received his Ph.D. in Psychology and Holistic Health from the University for Humanistic Studies in San Diego, CA. In 1971, as a member of the Peace Corps, he taught high school and junior college chemistry in Malaysia. He has been a health educator, professional consultant to individuals and corporations, and is a frequent speaker for clubs, organizations, and professional conventions. Dr. Pelton has been a stimulating guest on numerous radio talk shows throughout the nation. He currently serves as Assistant Administrator of Hospital Santa Monica, a holistic health hospital in Rosarito Beach, Baja, Mexico.

Taffy Clarke Pelton has a background as a marketing consultant and sales representative. She currently manages Agua Caliente Valparaiso, a hot mineral springs, holistic health spa in Tijuana, Mexico, where she also lectures and teaches aerobics classes. She is presently enrolled in a master's degree program in Psychology and Holistic Health at the University for Humanistic Studies.

Taffy and Ross, a husband-and-wife team, live together in Rosarito Beach, Baja, California. They strive to be a vibrant example of what they teach. Health is the major part of their lives and they have made a life-long commitment to helping others through health education.